PSYCHO-LOGICAL

Dean Burnett is a neuroscientist, blogger, author and occasional comedian. He lives in Cardiff. He is currently an honorary research associate at the Cardiff University Psychology School and a visiting industry fellow at Birmingham City University. He is an ambassador for the mental health charity Rethink and has received the Public Engagement of Neuroscience Award from the British Neuroscience Association. His books, *The Idiot Brain* and *The Happy Brain*, were international bestsellers and published in over twenty countries. His *Guardian* articles have been read over sixteen million times and he currently writes the 'Brain Yapping' blog for the Cosmic Shambles Network.

PSYCHO-LOGICAL

Why Mental Health Goes Wrong
– and How to Make Sense of It

DEAN BURNETT

First published in paperback by Guardian Faber in 2021
Guardian Faber is an imprint of Faber & Faber Limited
Bloomsbury House, 74–77 Great Russell Street, London WC1B 3DA

First published in audiobook by Audible in 2019

Guardian is a registered trademark of
Guardian News & Media Limited
Kings Place, 90 York Way, London N1 9GU

Typeset by Typo•glyphix, Burton-on-Trent, DE14 3HE
Printed in the UK by CPI Group (UK) Limited, Croydon, CR0 4YY

A CIP record for this book is available from the British Library

ISBN 978–1–783–35233–3

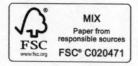

MIX
Paper from
responsible sources
FSC® C020471
FSC
www.fsc.org

10 9 8 7 6 5 4 3 2 1

Contents

Introduction

Hello, I'm Dean Burnett, and this is *Psycho-Logical*, a book all about mental health.

Now, mental health is a very big area, and a sensitive, evocative and emotional one at that. So, let's clear up a few things from the start.

Firstly, this is a book about mental health, but it's not about *my* mental health. No, this is a more general exploration of the current scientific understanding of mental health, covering what we think is going on in our brains (and sometimes bodies) when our mental health goes awry, why mental health problems are so common, and how people deal with all this and still live relatively normal lives. It's an as-logical-and-rational-as-possible look at psychological problems, hence the vaguely clever title.

The reason I don't talk about my *own* mental health is that I really don't have anything to say about it. Thus far, I've been one of the lucky ones who's never really had to deal with any difficulties with it. I've had my ups and downs, sure! I've encountered the extremes of the emotional spectrum thanks to things that have happened in my life, good and bad. But I'd say that these fall within the normal parameters of every-day human existence, as I've never been in therapy, taken psychoactive medication, or struggled to function in the wider world for reasons beyond circumstance, inexperience or just general ignorance.

Some people may be surprised to hear that, as pretty much any modern book about mental health focuses on the experiences of the author in dealing with their own issues. Obviously, I can't do this – at least, not without straying far outside of the non-fiction category. So, what gives me the right to throw my proverbial hat into the ring?

Well, let me begin by introducing myself. As stated, I'm Dean Burnett. I'm the author of *The Idiot Brain*, *The Happy Brain*, *Why Your Parents Are Driving You Up the Wall and What To Do About It*, and countless blogs, articles and other pieces of work centred around the quirky and weird properties of the human brain. I write about the brain because I'm a doctor of neuroscience. My PhD thesis is available at the British Library or the Cardiff University website if you want to check it out yourself.*

I was also head tutor and lecturer for Cardiff University's Masters course in psychiatry for many years, responsible for teaching qualified students and medics all aspects of psychiatry, from the basic science to the latest diagnosis and treatment methods, the rules and regulations governing their use, and much more. A job like that, coupled with years spent studying the workings of the brain itself, will certainly give you a very thorough understanding and appreciation of mental health and all the related aspects. Or so I'd argue, anyway.

Since then, I've written a lot about mental health, and people seemed to really like it when I did. A lot of things I've

* For the record, I don't recommend this. It's hardly a page-turner, unless you're really into the intricacies of whether the hippocampus is involved in retrieving memories for complex scenes and contexts.

written are now used as training, reference and teaching materials, by groups as diverse as A-level psychology courses, NHS libraries, organisations like the Samaritans, counselling bodies, and so on.

Why me, though? I'm not actually certified to diagnose and treat mental health problems, and there are undoubtedly thousands whose knowledge of mental health rivals or exceeds my own. So, why would I get singled out?

Well, I'm a neuroscientist for one. If it helps, think of me as an experienced car designer; I can tell you all about how cars work, but I can't necessarily fix yours, and I certainly can't issue you with a driving licence. Those are different skill sets.

I focus largely on the workings of the brain, and that's the one constant in all matters of mental health. You can't have mental health without the brain being involved, and it's a thing we can (within reason) look at, measure and analyse with science. By sticking to what's going on in the brain, I can hopefully make matters of mental health more grounded and relatable.

Also, I'm told my way of talking about mental health resonates because it's a lot clearer and more compassionate than most. Flattery this may be, but I will say that I do try to avoid inflexible conclusions and a hectoring tone, I endeavour to avoid stigmatising at all costs, and I always try to point out my own ignorance and the limits to my knowledge, so much so that my editors regularly ask me to stop.

Part of this tendency comes from the fact that I've been doing stand-up comedy as a hobby for close to twenty years now. Spending nearly two decades standing in front of drunken strangers who have no reason to like you, and trying to win them over in five minutes using just words, will patently affect your communication skills. It forces you to at least try to be relatable, likeable, engaging and comprehensible very quickly, or you get eaten alive.

I don't mean that literally, of course. Although you hear stories about certain gigs . . .

Perhaps a more important aspect was my upbringing, which differs greatly from that of most high-profile academics. I grew up in a pub, in a small dead-end South Wales former mining valley. I'm not having a pop at my childhood home of the Garw valley here – it's *literally* a dead end. There's no through road; it's basically a massive cul-de-sac.

It wasn't a hard or traumatic life by any means. But mental health is heavily influenced by environment, so if you grow up in a drinking establishment in an isolated, impoverished working-class village, you get to become very, shall we say *familiar* with a lot of mental health problems. And these people were my friends, my community, my extended family. It would be difficult for this not to affect your outlook on all matters mental-health-related.

In many ways, my learning about mental health later in life was like someone who grew up in the jungle doing a zoology course, being given a textbook full of familiar plants and animals and saying, 'Oh, *that's* what they're called.' I'd seen a lot of this stuff before; I just didn't have the vocabulary to describe it.*

* I also like to use analogies a lot, just so you know.

I promise I don't usually begin a book with an extensive complimentary profile of myself and my qualifications. But it's important to do that here because the modern world is, unfortunately, not short of people who like to lecture and harangue others on all matters mental health, despite having zero qualifications or even experience with the issues. If you've ever opened up about mental health problems of your own, you've almost certainly experienced this, having someone breezily telling you just to cheer up, or go for a run, or snap out of it, or think positively, or something like that. Or they'll tell you how you don't need medications because it's all a scam, or it's all in your head – like that's some breathtaking insight, rather than a statement of the thunderingly obvious. It's like telling someone with arthritis that it's all in their joints.

Even if their often unsolicited advice is one hundred per cent well meant – and that's something I remain sceptical about – such people invariably make matters worse. So, I want to make it abundantly clear that, for all my faults, I'm definitely not one of them. Because we're dealing with a subject matter that's very sensitive and deeply personal for millions of people. We're not talking about car tyre manufacturing methods here, or the agricultural policies of seventeenth-century mainland Europe.*

Of course, it's basically impossible to be one hundred per cent objective and rational about mental health. Therefore,

---

* That last one was something we covered in depth during my A-level history lessons, for some reason.

5

I'll probably still say things in the coming chapters that people will strongly disagree with or disapprove of. Apologies in advance if that happens. But at least now you're aware of the perspective from which I'm approaching all this.

So, that covers why I felt I could write this book. Now, why did I *want* to? What am I hoping to achieve here?

Well, it's probably safe to assume that you, dear reader, are reasonably aware already of mental health and matters associated with it. I base this conclusion on the fact that you're currently voluntarily reading a book all about this subject.

But consider how big a deal mental health awareness is in the modern world. We have World Mental Health Day, and many individual countries hold a Mental Health Awareness Week (or Month) every year. As well as this, there are countless books, copious websites, blogs, documentaries, and more. And that's not even counting the dedicated charities and organisations expressly set up to help people deal with mental health matters and learn more about them. We even have big-name celebrities opening up about their struggles and experiences. So, yes, raising mental health awareness is a big thing in present-day society.

To be clear, I support these efforts one hundred per cent. Much of my career has been about achieving exactly this. However, step back a second and ask yourself, how *effective* are these efforts at raising mental health awareness?

One answer to this is: very. In the past decade, I've noticed dramatic shifts in the discussion around mental health. It's now very common, for example, to see angry exchanges about whether or not antidepressants are valid treatment for depression, whereas not too long ago you were more likely to see people arguing that depression isn't a thing *at all*. So obviously, this awareness drive has been doing something right, even if there's still far to go.

But here's my main concern: awareness is great, but awareness does not automatically result in understanding. A lot of the time, campaigns and efforts impart a surprisingly simple message, amounting to little more than, for example, 'Depression is real – pass it on.' For the record, this statement is completely correct, but there are still people out there who believe otherwise. Unfortunately, the human brain is often quite a stubborn organ, meaning that if you want to change someone's beliefs, it requires more than simply telling them they're wrong.

Granted, you might say it's not just one person saying mental health problems are real, it's millions, and that's bound to be more persuasive, right? Quite possibly. But then, there are over a billion Christians in the world, a lot of whom are very vocal about their beliefs. And yet, atheists still exist.

Part of this is the fact that the human brain is more responsive to tangible, visceral experiences than it is to abstract, theoretical information. You can spend weeks learning dull material about, say, seventeenth-century European agricultural policies, and promptly forget it all once the exam is over. But you'll never forget your first kiss, or that terrifying car accident. Similarly, you can be told repeatedly that mental health problems are a genuine concern and never truly accept it, but if your *own* mental health encounters serious problems, then you know it's for real.

7

Think of all the complex systems that are omnipresent in the world around us, like cars, smartphones, plumbing, internet, the electrical grid, and so on. We're often utterly dependent on these things for our everyday existence, but how many of us actually know how any of them work? How many of us even give them a moment's thought, as we go about our daily lives?

The moment our car or central heating stops working, though, we're straight on to Google to look up timing belts and thermostats and whatnot. Because now it's a *problem*, so we're motivated to know what's going on.

This makes sense, in a way; our brains have finite resources to deploy moment to moment, so we're always more concerned with the things that seem more pressing and potentially hazardous than things that are familiar and reliable. So, if something's working as it should, we feel we don't need to know exactly how it works, just that it does.

The thing is, your mental health is even more integral to your life, and a great deal more complicated, than all the examples I just mentioned put together. Understanding it is a lot of work, and nobody's quite managed to get entirely to grips with it yet. So, perhaps it's to be expected that most people will prefer not to worry or even think about it. Unless their own mental health suffers in some way, that is.

And this brings me to another potential issue with the whole awareness aspect of the mental health debate. If we accept that the most effective way for people to be made aware of mental health is to experience issues themselves – because everyone has mental health, but not everyone has mental health problems – consider the following: one of the most widely cited statistics in efforts to raise mental health awareness is that one in four people in the UK will experience a mental health problem each year.

One in four.

Twenty-five per cent of the population!

Assuming it's accurate,* that's over 16 million individuals who experience mental health problems, each and every year, in the UK alone. A quarter of the country is acutely aware of mental health and what can go wrong with it.

If this is the case, why do we need to campaign for awareness at all? And why is it often such an uphill struggle? Why is it still a poorly understood and taboo subject, so often evoking paranoia and stigma? Fewer than one in four people support a football team of some description. And yet football is omnipresent, with rolling media coverage on all possible platforms, and nobody thinking it weird that the best players are worth more money than small countries.

If awareness of mental health is all that's needed, it should technically be as accepted and prominent as football, maybe with the best psychiatrists and therapists being traded between top hospitals for eye-watering prices.

Clearly, that isn't the case, so there's something else amiss when it comes to mental health. There are countless factors at work here, but I'd contend that it refers back to what I said just now: people tend to be more fearful and suspicious of

---

* And there is debate over this. But nobody denies that mental health problems are extremely common.

things they don't understand. The human brain really isn't a fan of uncertainty; it finds it unsettling by default.[1] And as useful and necessary as mental health *awareness* is, it doesn't automatically equate to mental health *understanding*.

Because mental health is regularly so much more intangible and harder to pin down in comparison to physical health, you need to do more than just insist it's a thing to convince people who've never experienced it to take it sufficiently seriously. Making people aware of something is only part of the battle. For instance, many people are *aware* that deep-fried food is bad for you, but they still keep eating it. Being aware of something doesn't automatically mean you do anything about it.

Perhaps if people had a bit more information, a bit more knowledge, a bit more understanding about exactly how and why mental health problems occur, we'd have more luck getting them acknowledged and accepted? And that's where this book comes in. This is my attempt to increase mental health understanding, not just awareness. I figured it's worth a shot, at least.

To help ground the issues in something more tangible, we'll be covering what's going on – or what we *think* is going on, according to the evidence we have – in the brain, when someone's mental health lets them down. We'll be looking at just how easy and commonplace these occurrences are, to help explain why mental health is such an issue for so many people. And, where possible, we'll be looking at how people experience and deal with mental health concerns and still live typical lives – because if one in four of us is dealing with some kind of mental health problem, the majority are clearly doing an excellent job of blending in with the rest of society. It's almost as if they're normal people. Imagine that!

It's also worth pointing out that even this impressive stat may be an underestimate. By the time this book comes out, the world will have been dealing with the global COVID-19 pandemic for over a year. Lockdowns, isolation, economic carnage, upended social norms and fraying international relations are just a few examples of the immensely stressful things abruptly inflicted on our civilisation. One very likely outcome of this, which is already starting to become apparent as I type this, is a marked increase in mental health problems, as countless people's lives are altered drastically, invariably for the worse.

This is especially true for me. In March 2020, my otherwise healthy fifty-eight-year-old father contracted COVID-19. In April, he died. I had to deal with that harrowing experience while cut off from my family and friends. The most traumatic experience of my life to date was one I had to come to terms with alone. Did this affect my mental health and emotional well-being? Undoubtedly. I can't see how it could have been otherwise.

My own knowledge of neuroscience and mental health has been useful, though. While it's not prevented the negative impact of such a painful experience, it's helped me understand how and why what's happening to me is happening. This has provided some reassurance and helped me cope with it all. Sadly, the enormous numbers of people out there who've gone through what I've gone through, and worse, won't have my existing and reassuring understanding of how all this affects our brains and our mental health. This book is my attempt to share what I know, in case anyone else might find it useful.

Also, despite the undeniable knock my own mental health has taken, thus far it's held up OK. I haven't needed therapy, or intervention from mental healthcare professionals. So, as well as sharing my own brain-based understanding, this book includes insights from people who have experienced, and had various forms of help with, serious mental health issues of their own – from actors and comedians to sex bloggers and teaching assistants.

At heart we are a social species, us humans, so it's often the case that hearing how other people have gone through things we're going through, or even just gone through things we're *worried* about, can be significantly more informative and re-assuring than any amount of meticulous but emotionally sterile research and evidence. And on a personal level, I think it's vital to include the perspective of those who've experienced the things I'm talking about if I've never directly dealt with it myself. Otherwise I'd be another one of those guys who thinks everything he says is automatically valid just because he's an educated straight white man with a media profile. And quite frankly, we've got plenty of that sort knocking about as it is.

Now let's get to what this book is all about: taking a calm and rational look at mental health, and all the associated difficulties it can lead to, in an effort to increase understand-ing and decrease suspicion and stigma. A logical approach to psychological problems. A Psycho-Logical perspective, if you like.

It would justify the title, at any rate.

1: The state of play

Mental health. What's that all about?

You might think this is a bit of a dumb, clueless question. Nevertheless, it's one this first chapter hopes to answer.

It's my plan, in this book, to look at some of the more common and recognisable mental health problems that people experience. I'll explore how and why they happen, what can be done about them, how these therapeutic approaches work, why they sometimes *don't* work, and anything else I can throw into the mix that might help explain what mental health is 'all about'.

Before we begin, let me clarify something that I *won't* be covering in this book.

Many people have valid complaints about mental healthcare services. Long waits for appointments and treatments, mixed messages, over-reliance on drugs, dismissive attitudes, even abuse and poor treatment at the hands of staff ostensibly charged with their care. These are all genuine problems that should be getting a lot more attention.

However, most of these can be blamed on politics, ideology, scarce resources, or just humans being unpleasant because they can, which is depressingly common. They suggest an ignorance or dismissal of mental health, *not* that the science underpinning it is wrong. It's like how the often-criticised UK railway network is the result of poor planning and bad management; it doesn't mean that the physics and engineering of locomotion need overhauling. It's a problem of application, not understanding.

So, please don't think me ignorant or dismissive of these matters. But, while I may touch on them where particularly relevant, they're not the focus of this book. I'm looking at the science and theory of mental health, not the flawed ways in which this information is often used.

OK, is that all clear? Good.

Now, let's get something else straight from the get-go.

Given the sensitivity of the subject matter, it's virtually guaranteed that I'll end up saying things here, making observations or claims, that some people will disagree with, possibly to the point of genuine rage or distress. I can only promise that this is absolutely not deliberate. I'm hoping to stick to the basic data and evidence we have, but I'm just one person, with small children and other obligations. I don't have the time, the resources, or the lifespan to absorb literally all the available information that humankind has produced about mental health. Therefore, I'm inevitably going to miss things, or misinterpret things, or just get things wrong.

The thing is, mental health, as a subject matter, is big, baffling, scary and complicated. And it will remain that way if you try and take it all on at once. That's why I focus largely on the brain. It's a better approach, to find one common thread and, basically, pull. See if you can unravel the whole thing. Or, see how the simpler bit works, and build up the more complex picture from there.

And yes, I did just refer to the human brain, the most complex single object in the known universe, as 'simple'.

That should give you a good idea about how tricky a subject mental health can be.

That is part of the problem, though. Because it's so complicated, intangible and subjective, there are many different approaches and theories regarding mental health, and most don't match up. Psychiatrists and psychologists regularly disagree on how to deal with disorders, or whether they should be 'dealt with' at all. Campaigners dispute the tactics of other campaigners. Practitioners argue with the views of patients, and vice versa. The mainstream portrayal of mental health often contrasts sharply with the reality. And on and on.

That's actually why I thought my perspective would be useful. Because while I'm by no means the defining authority on any particular aspect, my experience puts me in a relatively unique position as a kind of 'Jack of all trades' of mental health, from the basic science to clinical practice to the media portrayals.

If it helps, think of mental health as a music festival, and this book as an access-all-areas pass – you won't necessarily end up with the skill or experience required to get involved with the performances themselves (which in this analogy are the different aspects of mental health overseen by relevant trained professionals or directly affected individuals), but you can wander around all the different stages and see what's going on with each one.

At the risk of pushing this analogy well past breaking point, before you go to a festival and enjoy the performances, you do some prep, some planning. You pack your bags, see what the weather will be like, pitch your tent, get the lie of the land, find the stages and toilets and food stalls, all that sort of thing.

That, in essence, is the purpose of this first chapter. If mental health is a festival, then this is the preparation: figuring out what things are where, and working out what you want to see, and when. It's an effort to summarise the current understanding of mental health, overall.

What are these numerous approaches and theories? Who really thinks what, and why? Before we look at specific disorders, it's important to look at the backdrop on which they occur, by which they are defined.

I may be focusing on the brain, but the brain is shaped by the environment, by the world in which it exists. And that's even more true for mental health, and our understanding of it.

Mental health: what's that all about?

Let's start with the absolute basics. What *is* mental health?

For me, mental health is the overall quality, capability and effectiveness of your mind, or psyche, or whatever term you prefer. Just as someone experiencing no ailments and getting regular exercise is said to be in good physical health, someone who handles all the psychological demands and burdens of modern life with no obvious problems is said to be in good mental health. Hopefully, most people would be fine with this definition.

Of course, health is a complex process. The human body is composed of bones and organs and tissues and nerves and all that, but when we talk about someone's physical health, we usually mean the current state of *all these things* as a whole.

Yet you don't need *everything* to go wrong with your body for your health to suffer. Lung infections, kidney stones or heart palpitations are issues where only one part of the body is causing trouble, but the individual experiencing them is still said to be in poor health overall. The whole system is cohesive, interconnected and interdependent. The physical health of our bodies is like the Musketeers; it's all for one and one for all.

Our minds are also composed of many different elements, like emotions, instincts, thoughts, responses, perceptions, assumptions, memories, attitudes, beliefs, and so on. Mental health is essentially how well all these things are working together as a whole.

If they're chugging along without any noticeable issues, fine. But if your perception starts showing you things that aren't there, or you keep remembering traumatic things, or things that didn't actually happen, or you demonstrate extreme attitudes that are illogical or harmful, or your emotional reactions to things become too severe, or stop happening altogether, then you, or those around you, will start being concerned about your mental health.

So, just as we all have bodies and physical health, we all have minds and mental health, right? That seems a fairly harmless and reasonable conclusion.

Obviously, you've got your usual cynics and provocateurs, dismissing talk of mental health purely to cause upset, or for the attention, or a simple refusal to accept that there's something they don't know about. However, the truth is, when most people say 'mental health', whether they're dismissing it or campaigning for awareness of it, they usually don't mean general mental health, but the idea that you can have, or be prone to, *poor* mental health, to an extent that it stops you functioning normally.

Basically, it's not mental health, but mental *illness* that people are referring to. This is the concept a disconcerting number of people struggle with. There's even a surprising number of clinical psychologists, therapists and related professionals who deny mental illness is a thing. We'll look more closely at this surreal situation later.

Now, more observant readers will have spotted that this is the first time I've used the term mental illness, despite that being what most people getting this book will be interested in reading about. That's not an oversight, I promise. I will be talking all about the many problems that occur with mental health. But there are reasons that I don't say mental illness unless necessary, many of which get right to the heart of much of the copious debate and disagreement around mental health.

So, what's the problem with saying 'mental illness'?

Many reading this may find it exasperating. After all, how much time and money has been spent on convincing people that mental illness is a real thing that should be taken seriously? And yet here I am, claiming we shouldn't even say it!

If that's your reaction, I sympathise. I once felt the same way. However, I've since heard numerous reasons why people don't like the term mental illness, and many of them make sense.

Maybe that's why it's more common to hear the term mental *disorder* rather than illness these days. But the term mental illness is still regularly used, and for many, that's a problem.

The problem stems from the fact that you can't really observe someone's mental health. They usually have to tell you about what's going on in their head. And for this, they must use language. Unfortunately, using everyday language to describe a complex issue like mental health can be like trying to fix a watch with a rubber mallet.

Words have meaning. And if you use words with the wrong meaning in situations where accuracy is important, that can have bad consequences. This is particularly true in the context of medicine and therapeutics: imagine if an X-ray machine kept showing dark spots in people's lungs, whether there was anything there or not. That machine would be scrapped before you know it. Unfortunately, you can't scrap a word.

Of course, the meaning of a word isn't a problem if everyone knows exactly what it means. And we all know what illness means. Except . . . do we?

My dictionary defines an illness as 'a period of sickness'. OK, fair enough. But then I looked up sickness, and it is defined as 'the experience of being ill', which is . . . somewhat unhelpful, if you want to know what these words mean.

Because words like illness are undeniably important for medicine. In the 1980s, Professor Marshall Marinker,* attempted to clearly define disease, illness and sickness as three separate 'modes of unhealth'.[1] Disease, he contended, is the

---

* An experienced and influential general practitioner, who died in 2019.

actual pathology, like the infectious virus, the cancerous growth, and the consequences caused by it, that result in harmful changes from the biological norm. Basically, disease is the actual physical thing that affects someone's health. That's why, in the world of neurology, you get Parkinson's disease, or Alzheimer's disease. These things have a well-known and recognisable biological cause that results in serious disruption in the brain, leading to distinct symptoms. Hence, they're *diseases*.

Illness, he argued, is the subjective experience of a disease, of poor health. You may have a disease, but you *feel* ill. The unpleasant sensations you experience because part of your body or mind isn't behaving as it should – the discomfort and pain and incapacity – are how illness is defined. Hence you can feel ill before anyone knows what's wrong with you. Basically, it's up to you, the individual, to determine whether you're ill or not, because you're the only one who knows what you're experiencing.

Finally, sickness, which Marinker says is the external and public mode of unhealth. It's the social role you occupy as someone with a disease and illness. What's expected of you? How should you be treated and supported by others? This is why we get a sick note from our doctor if we're unable to work. We often need the validation of others to prove we're sick. We can't just insist we are.

So, under Marinker's system, a disease is the actual health problem itself, illness is the experience of it, and sickness is the acknowledgement of it by the wider world. That's all relatively straightforward. Unfortunately, the reality is a lot more complex.

For instance, if someone's taking regular medication, without which they'd die, are they 'sick'? Many would say yes. But this description applies to diabetics, and asthmatics, the vast majority of whom live perfectly normal lives. Similarly, is somebody sick if they're HIV-positive? Forty years ago, this was tantamount to a death sentence, so the answer was obviously yes. But now? A cocktail of medications reliably reduces the virus to a negligible presence, meaning the individual doesn't feel ill in the slightest, and isn't incapacitated in any way. Yet many would still insist that they're sick.

And this just concerns known physical ailments. Predictably, this issue of who can, or should, be classed as sick or not is a huge part of the discussion around mental health. Still, even if you don't agree with them, Marinker's definitions seem to reflect a lot of modern-day usage, so they're a decent basis to work from if you're involved in medicine or similar.

Thing is, though, I can blather on about the specific medical definition of illness all I like, but that's only useful if everybody else sticks to these definitions too. Unfortunately, they don't. Many people use the words illness, sickness, disease and so on as interchangeable. So, for ease of understanding, let's say that illness just means unwell, or experiencing poor health.

Now, a lot of the consternation around the label 'mental illness' is tied up with the fact that the term 'illness' is far more commonly associated with physical ailments, things going wrong with the body.

So, you get a lot of people regularly pointing out that mental and physical illnesses are basically the same and should be treated as such. You might have heard people comparing depression to a broken leg, for instance. Or maybe you've seen those memes showing what it would be like if physical health problems were treated like we treat mental health ones? People in a car crash being advised to go for a run and get some fresh air. People with cancer or serious diseases being told to snap out of it. People in the grips of an asthma attack being urged to just change your frame of mind, and so on. The general gist is, we should treat mental health matters the same as physical ones, because they're equally serious.

However, there are also those who strongly disagree, arguing, with good reason, that in many ways mental and physical health problems really aren't the same, and that equating the two can have immediate and harmful consequences.

Here's my take on the matter: there are situations and contexts where saying mental illness is like physical illness can be very helpful, and also those where it can be very unhelpful. Different approaches are needed in different scenarios. Laughing out loud at someone's best-man speech is appreciated. Laughing out loud at their eulogy is not.

Let's look first at the instances when equating physical to mental health *is* valid.

How mental health *is* like physical health

In my experience, comparing mental health problems to physical ones and emphasising the similarities is useful, perhaps essential, when dealing with those who have little or no understanding, awareness or acceptance of mental health problems, but are open to learning. That seems to be the default target of many mental health awareness campaigns.

As stated earlier, mental health issues are largely subjective experiences. Other people can't easily see what's going on in your head. So, to convince someone that mental health problems are real things with real consequences, you invariably need to frame them within more tangible, and relatable, references and concepts.

There's rarely any deliberate ignorance or bias here; it's just how the human brain learns things. A person's understanding of the world, and everything in it, is built up over the many years of their development and experience. We're said to hold in our heads a mental model of how the world works. This is effectively the sum of all the knowledge, experiences, assumptions, beliefs, predictions, and so on stored in our brain, which we use to inform and guide our decisions and behaviour. It's constantly updated as new experience and knowledge is fed into the system as we go about our lives, because at no point does the human brain ever just *stop*.

However, this does mean our ability to understand things depends largely on our own experiences. If someone starts talking to you in a language you've never heard, you obviously won't understand them. But our brains evolved to look for patterns and familiarity, so if there are words or tones or inflections that you recognise, you can start to deduce some meaning from the noises you're hearing. It's the same with a complicated concept or subject; if you need

23

to explain it to someone with no prior experience or aware-ness of it, then you need to present it in terms they can identify with and relate to.

For instance, people often say 'the human brain is like a computer', which us neuroscientists have mixed feelings about, because there are many stark differences. But when all's said and done . . . what else is there in everyday life that performs multiple complicated functions involving storing and manipulating information? It becomes the obvious com-parison, largely by default.

There's a famous phrase in medicine coined by Dr Theodore Woodward in the 1940s: 'When you hear hoofbeats, think horses, not zebras.' The gist is that the more common explan-ation is more likely to be correct. So, if people are more familiar with physical ailments and health problems than mental ones, they're going to think of those when they hear words like 'ill-ness' and 'unwell' and so on.*

It's also substantially easier to recognise physical problems in others. Our bodies are far more visible and consistent than our minds. If you're five foot seven and bald today, that's what you'll be for the foreseeable future.

So, if you see someone leaking black fluids from various orifices, or maybe just coughing and sneezing relentlessly, you know that shouldn't be happening, that they need help. You can confidently say someone's got a broken elbow if their

* Of course, that saying doesn't quite fit this situation, because mental health problems are very common, maybe even as common as physical ones. It's just a lot harder to see or observe them directly. It's like if zebras were as common as horses, but also invisible.

arm is pointing the wrong way, because everybody knows what the right way is.

None of this usually applies to mental health problems, though. They can usually only be observed indirectly, via someone's words, behaviours and actions. Your average person is going to have much less direct experience with mental health matters. For instance, if you see a good friend for the first time in a week, and they're now covered in sores, or have turned green, you'd (rightly) assume that something was seriously wrong.

But if when you last saw them they were happy, and now they're noticeably melancholy, you'd probably think little of it. After all, people's moods change all the time for a whole host of reasons, so someone's outward mental state being different after several days is hardly worth commenting on. Sure, this change could be due to a mood disorder or some other mental health problem. It could just as easily be because they recently got some bad news. It appears the same to those looking on from the outside.

Even trained professionals struggle to determine precisely what's wrong with someone's mental health, so the average person is going to have a much tougher time of it. This is something all those people who readily provide armchair diagnosis from a distance would do well to remember.

Also, let's not overlook the great deal of history behind physical vs mental ailments. Even the ancient Egyptians and Romans had their own systems of medicine and complex theories as to what it was that caused physical illness. Yes, most of their notions were laughably wrong when viewed through the lens of modern medical understanding, but they clearly had no trouble grasping the *concept* of poor physical health. That the functioning of the human body can be impaired and does go wrong in a wide variety of interesting and unpleasant ways is something that's been accepted for thousands of years.

Not so for mental health. While ailments like 'melancholia' have been documented since ancient times,[2,3] very little was actually known or done about them. It's only more recently, when our understanding of the mind has increased dramatically, coupled with our impressive progress in reducing or eliminating many of the causes of poor physical health, that mental health concerns have come to the forefront.

Of course, mental health problems aren't a modern invention. They were undoubtedly always there alongside all the classical maladies – all the poxes and agues and plagues that we know about – but went largely unacknowledged. Although you do see hints and signs of them throughout history: what are visions, prophecies, demonic possessions etc., but people seeing or hearing things that aren't there, behaving in irrational or illogical ways, and so on?

People in ancient times had no vocabulary or experience to describe or recognise mental health problems, so defaulted to explaining them in spiritual, religious or mystical terms. So hallucinations became divine visions or prophecies from God, while erratic behaviours became possession by spirits, requiring the somewhat invasive treatment of drilling holes into the victim's skull. Even today, we still hear of people who are dealing with mental health problems being described as 'struggling with their demons'.

26

It's hard to see how this historical background wouldn't also contribute to the modern stigma and suspicion around mental health. Centuries of potentially being burned at the stake or having your skulled prised open if you revealed mental health problems would surely have lasting consequences.

However, we live in a more rational and scientific world now, so such fantastical assumptions are no longer the norm. Instead, our go-to understanding is often based on physical health matters, and these are the terms and concepts often used to describe mental health issues as a result.

An optimistic stance would be that we're slowly moving to a point where mental health is more widely acknowledged and integrated into everyday language. Terms like mindfulness and well-being are now very familiar, and you often hear people referring to 'spoons', an increasingly common metaphor for the energy available to a person for the duties of daily life – for example, 'I don't have enough spoons for this today.' The spoons metaphor, coined by Christine Miserandino in 2003 in her essay 'The Spoon Theory',[4] can be used by those dealing with either physical or mental drains on their energy and motivation, so it's a useful term all round when talking about health.

Still, the language we have available remains somewhat limited when it comes to talking about mental health. Maybe we could create a whole new vocabulary, full of original terms to describe mental health and all that's associated with it? That would clear up all the uncertainty.

But then you'd need to teach that vocabulary to everyone in society, so that they know what it means. A daunting task, but if you don't do that, then introducing a whole new terminology will reduce understanding and awareness, not increase it. You're not going to persuade or educate anyone about anything if you start spouting unknown technical jargon, like an engineer from *Star Trek*. You'll just baffle them.

And there's one final point in favour of comparing mental to physical health issues, and it's the most straightforward. Put simply, there genuinely *are* many similarities between mental health and physical health problems.

Both mental and physical problems can manifest in a ridiculously large variety of ways. Both can be caused by a single traumatic incident, or build up gradually due to no obvious single cause. Both can be chronic, or fleeting. Both can range from relatively mild to completely incapacitating. Both can often be controlled or alleviated with regular medication or other therapeutic interventions. Both can have symptoms that come and go, persist all day every day, and everything in between.

However, despite these similarities, a common complaint about comparing the two types of problems is that physical health issues provide more certainty than mental health ones, so there are unfair expectations and assumptions about mental health problems conveyed along with the comparison.

This is often true, but it's worth remembering that physical ailments can also be subject to the same confusion and uncertainty that mental health ones are. I know someone who was taken to hospital with abdominal pains, and was told it could be constipation, a cyst, an infection, or kidney stones, all within a couple of hours. It's common to have a physical condition go undiagnosed for a very long time, or for a diagnosis to change repeatedly as more information about it is gathered.*

The human body is an incredibly complex system, and most symptoms are very far downstream from the actual cause, so trying to identify the cause of physical symptoms can often be like tasting wine and trying to work out the shoe size of the person who stomped the grapes.

Undoubtedly, this is a substantially bigger issue for mental health problems. But it's still a regular feature of poor physical health. Therefore, arguing that physical health matters are always straightforward is unfair and inaccurate.

So yes, overall there are plenty of ways in which mental and physical problems are very similar. Add to this the fact that your average person will be far more aware of, and have more experience of, physical illnesses, things that have been recognised and accepted for most of recorded history, and you can see why there are many occasions when saying mental health problems are like physical ones is the right thing to do.

How mental health is *not* like physical health

Having said all that, there are plenty of ways in which mental and physical health problems are NOT the same. There are copious differences in how they occur, how they work, and

---

* That's basically the format of every episode of the TV show *House, M.D.*, starring Hugh Laurie, practically the most popular show in the world for a period in the late noughties.

how they affect us. These differences can be, and often are, crucially important.

From certain perspectives, saying poor mental health is like poor physical health is akin to saying a frog is like a dog. After all, they're both common animals, have similar names, both have four legs and two eyes and a mouth. So yes, it's reasonable to say a frog is like a dog. Especially if you found yourself in a surreal situation of having to explain the concept of a frog to someone who's only ever seen dogs. Then you probably *would* describe frogs as small, wet, green dogs.

But if the person you were talking to then got themselves a pet frog, took it home, kept it in a nice warm basket and fed it dog biscuits, they'd quickly end up with a dead frog. Because in critical ways, a frog is *not* like a dog, and shouldn't be treated the same.

The main issue, both with this daft example and in the serious matter of mental and physical health problems, is that focusing solely on similarities while ignoring differences leads to limited understanding, and even harmful outcomes.

As mentioned, many would say that physical illness follows a predictable pattern: illness is confirmed, treatment is given (if one is available), person recovers and goes back to normal. That's the ideal, at least. It may be that the real picture is a lot more complex and uncertain, but 'treatment' or 'cure' are words commonly used in this situation. There's something that can be *fixed*.

But while physical health problems can often be cured or

repaired, mental issues are often more about adapting, coping, adjusting and managing. And some people find rather intriguing ways to cope. Here's a first-hand example of that, from the teaching assistant, comedian and storyteller Dan Mitchell.

I do find having a dog has helped me immensely, because the fact is, she doesn't understand the pressure, or all of these mood things. She just wants me to be happy. She doesn't judge, she doesn't do anything, but I have to take her out for a walk every day. These things I have to do because none of it's her fault. Having no children, I can only imagine it'd be a similar thing. Like having a child, there's something that depends on you, and therefore you have to push yourself to a certain extent. She does help me massively, and also, she is very amusing.

A dog needs to be walked. The walk happens no matter what mood I'm in. If I'm depressed, I don't want to do anything. Taking the dog for a walk, even with the depression, I might still wallow for the rest of the day, but I won't feel as if I haven't achieved anything. I will feel that I have at least done something. The dog is happy and she'll happily snuggle up with me then for the entire day if wanted, and I don't feel as bad about me. In the past, if I'd had a bad day with depression, I'd do nothing. Then I'd feel guilty about that, so I'd have another bad day the next day, which meant I'd do nothing again. It's a perpetual thing, you don't have the motivation to do anything, but you feel worse and worse for doing nothing. That one little thing, taking the dog for a walk, can make a difference to the next

31

*day, even if it doesn't make much of a difference on that
one day. It helps break the cycle.*

You hear many reports like Dan's, about how a key factor in
something like depression is staying active, keeping going,
even if it's only in minor, token ways. These are all useful
approaches, but the point is, you don't necessarily 'get rid'
of the problem; you find workarounds and ways to cope.
As a result, saying mental health problems are the same as
physical ones, or use of the word illness, leading people to
think mental issues work the same way, can imply an unfair
degree of certainty, predictability and fixability, something
mental health problems reliably lack.

That's a concern, for various reasons. If you suffer a mental
disorder for the first time and have been led to believe they
work like physical health problems, you may be expecting a
fix. But you almost certainly won't be getting one. Dealing
with poor mental health is difficult enough without the dis-
appointment and anger that stems from having your hopes
and expectations dashed.

Similarly, and more worryingly, convincing the wider
world that mental health problems are like physical ones
can make it *harder* for them to be accepted, not easier.
If you're someone who struggles with your own mental
health, have you ever had someone ask if you're better yet?
Or back to normal? Or be surprised when you have *another*
episode? Or get frustrated because they thought you'd dealt
with your problems? If this or similar has happened to you,
you've seen the negative consequences of people thinking

mental health works just like physical health.

Those who've had to take time off work for mental health reasons will be keenly aware of all this, unless your employer is extremely progressive and up to date, which is sadly still rare. There are numerous hoops you must jump through when taking time off work for health reasons, like set times before having to come back, or requiring sick notes or other forms of proof. Most of these were designed with physical illnesses in mind. They're a lot harder to manage when your health problems are mental in nature. Making someone with mental health problems jump through these hoops can be like forcing a dolphin to herd sheep. It's impractical, unreasonable, extremely difficult, and inevitably achieves nothing.

And if you're self-employed, it can be a big problem in other ways – an experience that freelance journalist Rachel England knows only too well:

> *My depression can be quite debilitating because I work from home*, I freelance. Getting up in the morning can be very challenging, because I don't have to be anywhere. I don't have to show my face at a certain time. Obviously, the joy of freelancing is that you set your own schedule. I'm naturally a very organised and disciplined person, so I'm grateful that my condition has never actually prohibited me from meeting deadlines and knowing what I need to do, but it does mean that the simple act of doing those things is massively exacerbated.*

---

* Something far more common at present, thanks to the pandemic.

I have a couple of regular clients, for example, who expect certain things to be achieved by certain times during the day and I always manage to hit that, but it's always at the expense of other things. I get up late and I won't shower because the idea of getting up ten minutes early to get in the shower just seems overwhelmingly difficult, too much of a challenge. Or eating, I feel like I haven't earned the right to eat breakfast until I've completed the duties that I need to do for the day.

Then, of course, all of that manifests itself in a greater impact of depression because then it's two o'clock in the afternoon and I've sat there in my pyjamas and I've not eaten anything yet, and none of that is conducive to a healthy body or mind.

Another issue is that with physical problems you tend to remain *yourself*, at least insofar as interactions with others are concerned. You may have a wretched cold or a broken leg or even a mystery illness, but you can talk about it as a separate thing, and social contact, where possible and safe, is usually a welcome distraction from your health woes. Hence hospitals have visiting hours.

But mental health problems *can* impact on your behaviour and interactions with others. Maintaining social interactions and norms can be hard work at the best of times, but it's even more taxing when you're in the throes of poor mental health.

The problem is, we humans put a lot of stock in social norms and pleasantries, so when someone starts behaving differently towards us, especially if it's a negative change, this can be very upsetting and cause lasting damage to a relationship. It's a sad fact that someone grappling with a mental health problem invariably needs more support and empathy than ever, but paradoxically, providing this support and empathy can often feel like a thankless chore to those who give it, because the person in need is not currently able to reward, thank or acknowledge them as we would normally expect. Consequently, relationships can be soured and compromised, just when they're at their most important.

This rings particularly true for the writer and actor Amelia Stubberfield, for whom the tolerance of others is a seemingly crucial coping mechanism . . .

I've had a lot of diagnoses, like depression, and anxiety, and most recently bipolar disorder. For me, the main thing that I experience is that my inner critic is massive. I have a constant and ongoing narrative in my head which is not even just critical, but actually actively quite bullying and very negative. I think that impacts, as you can imagine, on everything. I guess for me, it's the inner critic and this constant, pensive voice which leads to me trying to run away from my feelings by thinking my way out of it. Which doesn't work, obviously, and then that leads to anxiety.

I did have some very useful cognitive analytic therapy, where I discovered that, because of my early experiences where I found things very overwhelming, I'm almost needing people to hold my emotions for me and tolerate them for me, because I don't feel I can. But obviously no one can do that for you. I think the problematic or default

*coping mechanisms which evolved earlier on have been
to have that heavy reliance on external validation, which
probably does explain my acting career.*

*I have managed to establish and maintain some rock-
solid friendships; people I can just call up out of the blue
and say, 'I'm having trouble, I need help.' And they can do
that with me. It's usually the thing that keeps me going;
that gets me through it. It's so important to me and my
well-being to have that, and I think it's mutual with my
friends. But I'm incredibly lucky to have that, and it could
have been otherwise if I hadn't met the right people.*

That's just one example of how your interactions with others,
for better or worse, can be a crucial aspect of mental health.

Assuming that mental health problems are like physical
ones often completely ignores the possibility that the afflicted
person may think and behave differently to how they usually
do, hence it can take people by surprise and upset or frustrate
them, which usually makes matters worse.*

However, while all these drawbacks to comparing mental
to physical health problems are valid, there's one that gets to
the very core of much of the modern debate and conflict in
the area of mental health. How do you actually *confirm* when

---

* For a more concise and beautifully articulated summary of the problems with people conflating mental and physical health issues, check out
Hannah Jane Parkinson's exceptional *Guardian* article titled: "'It's nothing
like a broken leg": why I'm done with the mental health conversation.' It's
a pretty hard-hitting, emotional and sometimes harrowing read, so make
sure you're in the right headspace to deal with that before reading.

someone is mentally ill or unwell? Because before you treat someone for a health problem, it's important to confirm they actually have it. Nobody has open-heart surgery 'just in case'.

When we're talking about physical problems, it can be straightforward: a virus, a tumour, a deformity, a rupture caused by injury, a broken bone, and so on. These are all things we can detect and/or observe directly, thereby confirming that an individual's health is compromised. And even if we don't know exactly what the root cause of a physical illness is, the symptoms are often clear. We know how our bodies are supposed to work and what they should look like, so any drastic changes, particularly if they bring about pain and discomfort, are cause for alarm.

But there's no depression germ, or anxiety fungus. You can't have an overactive bipolar gland. The human mind is far more flexible, variable and changeable than the human body. It's also, you know, invisible. It very rarely expresses itself in ways that show up under a microscope.

How, then, do you determine whether there's something up with someone's mental state?

In fairness, sometimes it can be pretty obvious. Someone could experience mental issues that are clearly debilitating and distressing, to the extent they're totally unable to think, behave or function normally, maybe even putting themselves and/or others at risk as a result. That certainly can and does happen.

But it's also perfectly common for someone to have mental health problems and have them go unnoticed for a long time, even by the individual themselves. If we accept the statistic

37

that one in four people are dealing with mental health problems, most of them are clearly manifesting in ways that go largely unnoticed.

There's obviously a spectrum of severity with mental health problems, and it's important for us to know if and when to intervene, to offer help and support. So, at what point do we say someone has gone from mentally well to mentally *un*well? Where do you draw that line?

While this seems like another simple, straightforward question, it rarely is. It's one where many different groups have many different answers, many of which are incompatible, meaning there's no firm consensus on such an important matter.

There are those who insist that even mild deviations from normal mental functioning warrant medical intervention. There are those who insist that normal mental functioning is a totally meaningless concept, so medical intervention is never warranted. And there are various positions between these two equally alarming extremes.

The purest approach is, perhaps surprisingly, mathematical. It might seem odd to invoke maths in the arena of mental health, but it's not impossible. This approach is often used in abnormal psychology, a discipline dedicated to the study of unusual patterns of thought, behaviour and emotions, so obviously applies to mental health a lot.

Basically, if you assign a numerical value, a score, to a trait or type of behaviour, you can work out the average, the 'normal' score of a population, and anyone with a score that is too far off that norm, or mean, can be said to be *ab*normal, at least regarding the thing being measured.

The best example is IQ.[5] The average IQ of a population is 100. Always. That's how it works. There's a lot of complex maths involved, but if you do an IQ test and get a score that is more than 30 points off 100 (i.e. a score lower than 70 or higher than 130), you have an abnormal IQ, because of the way the distribution of IQ varies within a given population. And if you can score other traits and aspects of mental health in this way, you could presumably perform similar calculations.

The benefits of this approach are that there is, in theory, no judgement or ideology involved. It's just numbers. Having a below-average IQ is just as abnormal as having an above-average one. And while you may be able to argue with a personal assessment, it's difficult to argue with a calculation. It is what it is. Two plus two is going to be four no matter how you feel about the number four.

On the downside, this approach is seriously limited. It's often ludicrously hard, if not impossible, to apply a numerical, quantitative value to mental health properties. What's your exuberance score? What percentage anxious are you? On a scale of one to fifty, how would you rate your sense of ennui? How much does your motivation weigh? It's hard enough to do this with physical issues, like how patients are regularly asked to rate their own pain on a scale of one to ten, because there's currently no better way for clinicians to measure someone's physical discomfort.

Despite the constant efforts to impose consistent numerical values on how people think and behave, particularly in the corporate world, the human brain simply doesn't play ball there. It's like trying to nail down fog.

On top of this, while it technically *shouldn't* happen, there have been many instances in the past where ideology and prejudice heavily influenced such testing. In the early twentieth century there were notorious instances in the US of IQ tests suggesting many immigrant and lower-income adults had shockingly low IQs, with these results being used to justify a raft of exclusionist and oppressive policies. The problem wasn't the IQ of certain demographics, though. It was the tests, invariably created by wealthy white men with the privileged backgrounds that allowed someone to work in science in the early 1900s. The tests included questions that asked the subject to identify things like tennis courts and light bulbs, the sort of things poor people in 1910 would probably never have even heard about, let alone seen; bias was inbuilt.

Clearly, other approaches are needed when it comes to determining when someone is officially mentally unwell.

Maybe it's when they're experiencing genuine stress and discomfort due to what's going on their mind? This would apply to things that people find very debilitating, such as depression and anxiety. We saw earlier that medicine tends to think of illness as the personal experience of poor health. Essentially, mentally unwell people can say 'I need help', and that's when we know something's wrong.

However, it's often not easy to ask for help with mental health issues. It carries a lot of risk in a society where stigma is still rife, but the problems with openly saying you need help are different to being aware that you need it.

But perhaps a bigger problem with this approach is that there are many times when people with mental health problems aren't aware that anything's amiss. Our awareness is a facet of our mind, after all, and if our mind is compromised in some way, then our awareness could be too. People with dementia often passionately deny that there's anything wrong with their memory, even when talking to a close family member they don't recognise. People who are delusional or hallucinating frequently don't realise that's what's happening. They've been trusting their senses all their lives. Why would they stop now?

In cases like this, another approach is to assess whether the person's behaviour is maladaptive, meaning unhelpful or harmful. This can mean harmful to the health of the person afflicted – often labelled biologically maladaptive: the black moods or zero motivation of depression, or the incapacitating panic attacks of anxiety, or someone in the grip of paranoia who's harming themselves, or in a manic state engaging in thrill-seeking behaviour that could injure or kill them, and so on. In every case, a change has occurred, and it's affecting the individual negatively; therefore, it can be considered biologically maladaptive.

Alternatively, changes to someone's mental health can be *socially* maladaptive – harmful to others, or society overall – like an addict committing crimes to fund a drug habit, or someone with sociopathic tendencies actively hurting others because they don't see any reason not to. Overall, the logic goes that if someone's behaviour or mental state changes in ways that prove to be harmful to themselves or others, for no discernible rational reason, they can be confirmed as being mentally unwell.

So, someone's mental state may be statistically abnormal, it may cause them distress and/or impaired functioning, it may cause them to behave in ways that are harmful, to themselves or those around them, for no valid reason; put all that together, and you might think there's a decent set of criteria for recognising when someone has problems with their mental health. And much of the time, you'd be right.

Now, consider the following. It was only in 1973 that the American Psychiatric Association, the APA, declassified homosexuality as a mental disorder. Other mental health organisations did the same around the same time, by and large. So, fifty years ago (at the time of writing), if you were gay, you were officially mentally unwell. It's startling to realise that we went from classifying homosexuality as an official sickness to legalising same-sex marriage in under five decades. Sure, there are still plenty who feel homosexuality is sick and wrong, but for the most part these such views are no longer held by the medical establishment.* However, uncomfortable as it may be to consider, it's possible to argue that homosexuality *did* tick all those boxes I mentioned for a mental illness.

A minority of people in the population are homosexual, so it could be described as statistically abnormal. Sex is for reproduction, so any sexual activity outside of male–female intercourse is wrong and harmful, unnatural, therefore homosexuality is biologically maladaptive, damaging. And many

* In developed Western countries, that is. There are plenty of places where homosexuality is still deemed a crime, let alone a disorder.

homosexuals struggle with the stigma around their sexuality and the trauma and stress of coming out, or staying in, so it causes a lot of personal discomfort and upset. Again, biologically maladaptive.

And reproduction is crucial to sustain society, right? Homosexuality doesn't allow for reproduction, so is therefore socially maladaptive, harmful to society. Looked at this way, it makes logical sense to classify homosexuality as a mental disorder.

Except . . . we know it isn't one. At all.

Homosexuality is perfectly natural. It's observed in many species and has been around for as long as the human race. Only a minority of the population are gay, but a similar minority of people have red hair, and that's not been labelled a medical problem at any point. Plenty of people don't or can't have children for various reasons, but they don't warrant a mental health diagnosis. And the idea that human sexuality is solely about male–female reproduction is laughably naïve. We humans, like our bonobo cousins, use sex for a wide variety of purposes. Basically, human sex and sexuality are far more complex and varied than such narrow restrictions account for.

Here's the key point: homosexuality was once an official mental illness, and now it isn't. But homosexuality *never changed*; it was deemed to be a problem when measured against the societal consensus of what was normal and healthy. But that *consensus* changed. Our understanding and appreciation of sexuality expanded and developed. Society once concluded that something was wrong and immoral.

43

Then society changed its mind. It adapted, moved on, grew up. At least in part.

And there you have the crux of the matter. Physical illness is determined by physical norms, and physical norms don't change. The human body is relatively fixed. A Roman citizen's internal body temperature was thirty-seven degrees Celsius, just like ours, and a heart attack in the 1300s was the same as a heart attack today. We're very familiar with what the normal functioning of a human body is, and therefore can be very sure if something's gone or is going wrong.

The same cannot be said about mental health. Mental health problems are measured against mental norms, norms of thinking, norms of behaviour, norms of belief. And these norms *can* change, sometimes very rapidly. They're social constructs, and societies are constantly in flux. This leads to a great deal of confusion and inconsistency, making it ever harder to pin down poor mental health.

Consider the following: if someone regularly and knowingly consumes a poison, one that causes violent tendencies and damages brain functioning, and doesn't see any issue with what they're doing, are they mentally unwell? According to the criteria I've described, yes.

Unless it's alcohol, in which case it's fine. Standard behaviour.

If you're constantly talking to an invisible alien called Zobbo, who you say follows you everywhere, you're assumed to be hallucinating, or delusional. But swap Zobbo for God, an intangible superbeing responsible for all existence, and that's fine. Then you're not unwell; you're religious. People will praise your piousness. Do it often enough and they might let you live in the Vatican and give you a big hat.

And for many of those who criticise modern approaches to mental health, that's where concerns lie. The criteria we use to judge who's mentally well and who's mentally unwell are so malleable, so flexible. Who's to say that what we deem to be acceptable, helpful and proper practice today won't be condemned and vilified tomorrow? The homosexuality example is a perfect illustration. So-called gay cures are widely condemned and vilified for the serious harm they cause, but not too long ago those same methods were being used by extensively trained, officially qualified and regulated therapists.

It's important not to lose sight of such issues. We judge people's mental health based on social norms, but society is messy and confusing. You might see the mainstream coverage or online campaigns and conclude that everyone's cool and on board with mental health matters now, but sharing positive memes is not the same as society-wide acceptance. There are still many homes and communities where mental health is a subject barely even acknowledged, let alone accepted. Any individual growing up in such an environment with mental health problems will have a lot more to overcome as a result.

Wider society is far from perfect. Sexism, for example, is still a big problem, one with many consequences for mental health. Women were historically the most common recipients of lobotomies.[6] The world 'hysteria', meaning wild or excessive emotions, is derived from the Greek term for

45

uterus, because it was deemed something only women could experience. Indeed, a few centuries ago it was believed to be caused when the womb somehow detached and went wandering through a woman's body, causing disruption.*

You may also have heard the term nymphomania, to mean someone with an uncontrollable need for sex. But nymphomania is something only women could be diagnosed with. The male equivalent was called satyriasis, but that never entered common usage. I'd wager you've never even heard the term before now. Why not? One likely explanation is cultural double standards. A woman who wants a lot of sex? That's so unusual she must be ill, and needs medical intervention! A man who wants a lot of sex? That's not an illness. That's Tuesday. These are the norms.

We now use the term hypersexuality for either sex, and libido and arousal vary far more between individuals than they do overall between the sexes. But still, this is only a recent development, and default assumptions are still that men's sexual needs and drives are radically different from those of women.

Similarly, the general belief that women are overly emotional, and men are inherently stoic, harms both. The expectation that men be constantly strait-laced and strong and not show emotion is believed to be a big factor in toxic masculinity, and the fact that suicide is a major cause of death for young men in developed society,[7] where men aren't 'allowed' to express emotions.

---

* To clarify: internal organs literally never do this.

Guy Kelly is an actor and comedian who has written shows about this issue, and has some very firm views about it.

I think the reason male mental health is so often overlooked and underdiagnosed and generally leads to pub brawls and suicide is that feelings are seen as 'things that women have'. Society says that 'Women are other. They have feelings. Men are men. They have sex.'

That is a dichotomy that you can't cross. A woman doesn't want to have sex. A woman has sex done on her. A man doesn't have feelings unless he's bloody soft. It's a whole society change that needs to be made. This, 'Men don't cry. Boys don't cry. Man up. Be a man.' Women have the reverse of that: society at large has the common consensus, 'Women are emotional. They can't keep their emotions in check.' No. It's just that they're socialised to be more open with emotions. The outbursts that fucking Donald Trump has had, if it were a female person having those, it would be like, 'Oh. Shout it from the rafters about this hysterical woman!'

I'm still guilty of this. I'm more emotionally close with my female friends than I am with my male ones. I've tried. I reach out, and I do this, but I'm still more comfortable talking to women. I can only give as good as I get. I will have close and emotionally involved conversations with my male friends, but they're not the day-to-day people I contact.

That's weird and sad in the same way that it's sad that science has missed out on however many hundreds of years of female scientists. Who knows how emotionally acute and sensitive some of my male friends are. I've got a friend of mine who I've known since I was three. I was the best man at his wedding, he was the best man at mine. I don't think we've ever had a heart-to-heart.

That's obviously my fault as much as anybody else's, but you're sort of built into that. If the banks have been eroded in a certain way, the river finds it harder to fuck off elsewhere.

There are so many other cultural and societal factors that affect our understanding of mental health, but you get the point. To bring it full circle, this is perhaps the most important reason why many object to the term mental illness. If something's described as an illness, it is, by definition, something wrong, something that shouldn't be happening, something needing to be fixed. But there was a time when homosexuality was considered an illness. It clearly isn't. Treating it like one, and attempting to cure it, caused way more harm than just accepting it.

So, when you refer to a mental illness, you could be causing misunderstanding, introducing unfair and unhelpful expectations and assumptions, and even be asserting that there's a problem when there isn't one. Because maybe it's society that's wrong about how a person should behave and think, not the person themselves?

Basically, when the social norms and expectations that we measure people against can change so much, who has the right to say whether someone's mentally unwell, or not?

That's not a rhetorical question; an obvious answer would be doctors. Specifically, psychiatrists, in this case. Isn't that the whole point of medicine; to determine when someone's unwell and do something about it?

Luckily for pretty much everyone, medicine and science haven't just looked at the problems around mental health and promptly given up. Far from it. They've mostly acknowledged all these issues and done their best to incorporate or allow for them when researching how mental health works and figuring out the best approaches to dealing with the many problems that arise from it. So please don't think that everyone who works with mental health problems is just 'winging it'. Nothing could be further from the truth.

However, medical science and mental health have a complicated relationship, one that's increasingly important to acknowledge as our awareness of mental health evolves.

The pros and cons of the medical approach to mental health

What's the difference between a psychologist and a psychiatrist?

Yes, they do sound similar, but so do the words frog and dog, and let's not get into that again.

When you work in the field, it can be surprising to realise that many don't know the difference. I used to oversee a Psychiatry Masters programme, and many applicants said they had done a psychology degree because they wanted

49

to be a psychiatrist. It was always awkward, having to tell them that they'd made a terrible mistake.

I don't mean that being a psychiatrist is a terrible idea.* I mean that a psychiatrist, in the UK and US at least, must be a medical doctor, someone who's gone through medical school and is qualified to practise medicine. If you've done a degree in psychology instead, you can't be a psychiatrist. Those are the rules.

There are good reasons for this. Medical doctors have been tackling poor health for centuries, so when mental disorders were (finally) acknowledged as the legitimate health issues they are, they were inevitably incorporated into the established medical system. But it's not purely a matter of 'that's just how things panned out'. There are many practical reasons why psychiatrists should be qualified physicians.

Firstly, they frequently need to prescribe powerful medications, like antipsychotics, antidepressants, and more. Psychoactive medications shouldn't be given out freely to all comers, like sprinkles on an ice cream. They absolutely should be handled by trained professionals, just as aeroplanes should be handled by pilots. And you need a thorough understanding of human physiology if you're going to prescribe medications that have many significant biological effects.

There's also another matter, one that I've avoided thus far just to keep things simpler. Basically, physical and mental health problems aren't mutually exclusive. Quite the opposite. They go hand in hand, all the time.

* Although I've met some psychiatrists who wouldn't dispute that.

The brain influences the body and the body influences the brain, and problems with one regularly spread to the other. This can result in comorbidity, where different diseases or health problems occur at the same time, often due to the same cause. The human body and mind certainly don't operate a 'one-in, one-out' system when it comes to things going wrong.

But rather than infectious agents or injuries, mental health problems are often caused by traumatic life events and/or extremely stressful situations or circumstances. Therefore, it's hardly surprising that people with terminal cancer or dementia also regularly end up with a depression diagnosis too.[8] Learning that you have a fatal or incurable condition surely qualifies as a traumatic experience, as does dealing with it daily.

There's also the factor of mental health problems having physical causes, and vice versa. As well as traumatic events or psychological disturbances, many mental disorders are also linked to physical factors like genes, toxins, internal chemical balances, and so on. Accordingly, it helps greatly to have someone who knows about physical health when it comes to treating mental health. They take more variables into account, do extensive histories, know all the relevant tests, know what treatment options are available, and so on.

So yes, psychiatrists being as comprehensively trained in physical and mental health as a single person can be is a useful, often essential approach.

This is made possible by the fact that medicine has made many advances since the days of drilling holes in skulls. There have been centuries of case reports and studies and so on, all refining and expanding our knowledge of mental health. And this accumulated knowledge is readily available to those who need it, particularly those charged with tackling mental health issues. When it comes to recognising, assessing and diagnosing mental health disorders, the two main classification systems used by mental healthcare professionals are the Diagnostic and Statistical Manual of Mental Disorders[9] (aka the DSM) and the International Classification of Diseases[10] (aka the ICD).

These are distinct documents produced by different organisations, but both provide extensive and exhaustive details about all the officially recognised and catalogued manifestations of mental health dysfunction. There's a lot of overlap between them, as you'd expect (and hope). Both are extremely detailed and very large, given they cover all the disorders recognised by medical science, with added appendices to cover the issues that *might* be problems, but are still being studied. Both are used extensively in professional settings. And, in acknowledgement of both ongoing research and the shifting cultural standards I mentioned earlier, both are regularly revised and updated, to reflect our ever advancing understanding of mental health thanks to research, clinical reports, and so on.

At the time of writing, the DSM is on its fifth edition, the DSM-5, while the ICD is on its eleventh, the ICD-11. Remember when I said homosexuality was dropped as a mental illness? The DSM and ICD are what it was dropped *from*. Mental disorders and conditions are constantly being removed, added, reclassified, or otherwise moved around, as the available information and understanding of them develops.

Indeed, the ICD is predominately a coding system, where each disorder is given a specific sequence of codes, so clinicians can know exactly what they're dealing with. The ICD-9 used a five-digit numerical coding system, which allowed around thirteen thousand codes for specific disorders. Updating to the ICD-10 was deemed necessary when it was realised that this wasn't enough. The ICD-10 had a new alphanumeric coding system allowing for at least sixty-eight thousand codes!*

It shows how drastically our medical understanding has expanded in recent years when an official list of disorders arguably contains five times as many diagnoses as the previous version.

However, while the DSM and the ICD overlap substantially, there are key ways in which they differ. These documents essentially dictate the care and medical advice received by millions of people, so such differences are important.

I should remind people at this point that I'm not a practitioner or psychiatrist myself, so the following is based on my own research, not on any experience of using these systems in professional, clinical settings, which could make a big difference to how they're viewed.

The DSM is produced by the American Psychiatric Association, while the ICD comes from the World Health

---

* These aren't all for mental health disorders, of course, as the ICD covers all health problems, so most of these entries will be for more physical issues. But still, the range of mental health codes now runs to over 300, with many subtypes and subcategories, so it's still a notable expansion.

Organization. The DSM focuses solely on mental health, while the ICD covers *all* known health problems, with a section on mental health.

The DSM includes detailed descriptions of the disorders, to help clinicians recognise and manage them. The ICD is more about assigning a specific code to a disorder upon diagnosis, which is great for cataloguing, data gathering, and invoicing for the costs of treatment, but not so helpful when you actually want to know what to do about a disorder once it's been diagnosed.

Based on this, you may assume the DSM is the more useful system. It's produced by clinical practitioners *for* clinical practitioners, it's more detailed about how to recognise and deal with disorders, and has a narrower scope, in that it focuses solely on mental health problems rather than health overall. Indeed, many mental health practitioners defer to the DSM for these reasons.

However, the ICD has several advantages too. It's the work of the World Health Organization, based on accumulated data from 196 member countries. It is multilingual and produced by a not-for-profit organisation, so is free to access and use, with a view to helping all countries, particularly developing ones, to recognise and therefore reduce the burden of health problems in the population. It can be, and regularly is, adapted by the country using it to best fit their existing healthcare set-up.

The DSM, by contrast, is produced by an American organisation, so there's an inevitable cultural leaning. It costs money; the DSM-V was originally released at a cost of $199

– thus, it generates revenue for the American Psychiatric Association.

But the latest edition caused a lot of controversy for other reasons. Many objected to how standards of assessment for what warranted a medical diagnosis had been noticeably lowered,[11] so now things like tantrums in children[12] or grief in adults[13] are in the DSM and are therefore deemed psychological disorders, rather than normal emotional expressions of the developing or mourning human mind.

As ever, the details and specifics of these new inclusions into the DSM are more complex and nuanced than many of the impassioned arguments imply. Not *every* tantrum or experience of grief automatically becomes a mental health problem. Far from it.

But still, changes to diagnostic criteria like this have been made. Proponents of the DSM's approach and ethos, and those responsible for it, contend that these changes are necessary to address limitations and irregularities in existing understanding of mental health problems and their associated treatments, and to deal with the harm that this can cause.

There is indeed a case to be made here: for instance, excessive tantrums in certain children were often deemed as evidence of bipolar disorder, with powerful medications being prescribed to deal with it. With the addition of a specific disorder concerning tantrums, this is no longer necessary.

Some view these changes and expanded diagnoses as welcome acknowledgements of the omnipresence of mental health problems in our everyday world. Others, though, believe it shows something more cynical, like the unacceptable influence of capitalist interests (namely pharmaceutical companies) in the classification and criteria of mental disorders, thanks to their significant involvement in the US healthcare system. The new changes would logically result in more people being diagnosed and requiring medication, which is lucrative for those very same companies.

This understandably set off alarm bells for many. You may have heard of the medicalisation of normal human traits: that's what this is, bringing more and more relatively normal things under the umbrella of official health problems, so they can be 'treated'. The motivation might be profit, convenience, or a desire to ensure conformity. It's an ongoing concern, and something to be very wary of, particularly in light of the aforementioned problems with defining what does and doesn't count as a mental disorder.

This isn't a criticism exclusive to the DSM. The ICD drastically increasing the number of possible disorders it included was similarly seen as clear evidence of a drive to classify normal expressions of human diversity as medical problems. You may agree with this conclusion. Or, you may accept that it's more likely due to an overhaul of the classification system. That there are more than five times as many disorders in the latest version of the ICD compared to the previous one strongly suggests it's not just a matter of broadening the definition of what counts as a disorder.

But this isn't to say that there isn't a valid concern regarding over-medicalisation, or however you describe it. In 1989, researchers Stefan and McManus published a study[14] where medical students were surveyed on what ailments they considered to be diseases. Interestingly, those in the fifth year of medical training were far more generous with the disease label than those in the first or third year of medical school. Put simply, it reported that the more medical training someone has, the more likely they are to consider an ailment as a disease.

One particularly relevant result was that only twenty-five per cent of first-year medics considered depression a disease, while only twenty-five per cent of fifth-year medics thought depression *wasn't* a disease.

As we covered earlier, disease is a specific term, one that most mental health problems don't, or shouldn't, warrant. So, why would extensively trained medics think otherwise? And, given that they're so highly educated, maybe they're actually the ones who are right?

You could make this argument. Many do. But remember what I said earlier about how your experiences affect how you think, understand and perceive things? It's fair to say that the bulk of medicine is concerned with physical problems. Oncology, cardiology, haematology, nephrology, dermatology, immunology; there are many different medical specialities, but the majority deal with matters of the body. So, if you're repeatedly told, day in, day out, for several years about the physical issues that lead to health problems, why *wouldn't* you see every health problem as something with a physical cause, to be targeted and dealt with?

Except, mental health problems often can't be remedied in the same way as you would a physical ailment, as they have far more complex and intangible causes. And problems arise when doctors go ahead and try it anyway, which seemingly happens a lot.

This sort of approach is what's known as the medical model of mental illness.[15] It's sometimes called the disease model, for obvious reasons. It describes the practice of approaching and dealing with mental disorders as if they were physical problems, and mental health patients the same as any other type of patient.

We've already looked at why this can be a bad idea, but it was the go-to approach to mental health problems in medicine for many years. It often still is, but it's hopefully on the wane, with more holistic or nuanced approaches taking over that reflect the complex and multifaceted nature of poor mental health.

There are several problems with the medical model. One is that it assumes there's a clear and accurate diagnosis to be had, with a specific cause, specific symptoms, and a reliable prognosis. It also dictates that the patient assumes a passive role; they accept the diagnosis, do what the doctor says, and conform to their treatment regimen (usually some form of medication). They do this, eventually get better, and the process comes to an end.

These are the usual assumptions of the medical model. But the thing is, mental health problems regularly thwart all of them. They can seldom be pinned to a single physical cause, they manifest in such a mind-boggling (no pun intended) number of ways that a definite diagnosis is often elusive, and expecting someone not to get involved with what's going on in their own mind is quite a big ask!

For example, let's focus on the bit about needing a specific diagnosis. The DSM lists nine symptoms linked to depression,[16] such as a depressed mood for most of the day, disrupted sleeping patterns, feelings of worthlessness or excessive guilt, and so on. It then says a patient must display five of the nine symptoms, for a minimum two-week period, to be diagnosed with depression.

This means you could easily have two people with the same diagnoses, but only *one* of many symptoms in common. Depression is having almost completely different effects on them, yet they should be labelled and treated in exactly the same way? You can see why a lot of people aren't on board with this approach. As you might suspect, or hope, the process is much more complex than this. Psychiatrists don't just diagnose people according to simple checklists, they take copious other factors into account, otherwise anyone with a clipboard could do their job. But it hopefully shows that a reliable, specific and accurate mental health diagnosis is no easy task, given just how variable and intricate the human mind tends to be.

Then there's the assumption that the patient must take a passive role in the process. With physical problems, that makes sense; the doctor is the one who knows how the intricate mechanisms of the body work, what's going wrong, what the medication does, and the patient is expected to trust their expertise, in order to ensure the problem is dealt with effectively.

But even then, the patient often has a vital role in the recovery of physical problems, such as with physiotherapy.

Surely this is even truer for a mental disorder? It might be more efficient and straightforward for the healthcare system to keep patient contributions to a minimum, but when the only information you can glean about a problem comes from what the patient tells you, expecting them to remain quiet during the whole process is often counterproductive.

Overall, effective treatment of mental health problems usually requires more equality and balance in the patient–doctor relationship. But sticking to the medical model skews it drastically in favour of the latter, causing unnecessary obstacles. We've also covered the idea of 'getting better' with mental health problems, and why that's often not a realistic prospect, yet it's built in to the medical model, at least in theory.

So yes, modern medicine may have a great deal to offer the world of mental health, and regularly saves countless lives, but there are still issues and questions to be answered regarding its methods and approaches. Yes, it's identified a vast number of conditions and treatments, and is adding more all the time, for better or worse, so it's hopefully good to know mental health is taken so seriously by the relevant professionals. Nonetheless, many argue that focusing on specific clearly defined disorders is the wrong way to go about mental health.

There are good reasons in favour of it, in fairness. Most obviously, the fact that drugs are so often effective and useful. Drugs affect us on the fundamental biological level, and specific types and classes of drugs having beneficial effects on numerous conditions strongly suggests that there is indeed one common underlying factor or cause for such conditions. Therefore, specific diagnoses can be a valid approach.

It's sort of like how you can have a dozen cousins who look and act nothing alike, but they all share a set of grandparents, so you can't deny they're part of the same family. A diagnosis of a disorder can be said to work the same way; it can be expressed in a startlingly varied number of ways, but there's a common, often biological, thread to all of them.

I made a similar point earlier when I said I'm going to stick to what's going on in the brain because the bigger picture is too big and confusing, and it helps to narrow the focus. Because when explaining how mental health works, trying to take into account *every possible variable and factor* that affects it would, while being undeniably thorough, quickly end up being overwhelming and outright baffling. Hence, I've opted to stick to common themes and elements, rather than include literally everything. It's really the only way to get anything done. Better to tackle part of the problem and make progress than try to take it all on and get nowhere, right?

But why wouldn't the same apply to *treating* mental health problems? It would be churlish of me to call out the entire medical profession for methods I use myself.

As compelling as this logic may seem, though, many would argue that problems with mental health are nowhere near as logical and clear-cut as that.[17] Medics often end up trying to make the symptoms fit the diagnosis, rather than the other way around, while ignoring or dismissing any of the patient's input and insight that make this trickier. You basically end up with a constant effort to get many square pegs into more convenient round holes. Predictably, this causes a lot of friction.

The psychology perspective of mental health

A lot of that friction is between psychologists and psychiatrists. Now that we all know they're not the same thing, that might be alarming to hear. You'd assume that they'd be working together to tackle mental health problems, right?

Luckily, most of the time, they are doing just that, and it works out best for everyone. You can't have a football team where every player is a striker, after all.* Similarly, there are many ways in which the disciplines and approaches of psychiatrists and psychologists differ, so when they collaborate it leads to a wider range of options, perspectives, and methods for tackling mental health issues, giving those afflicted an even greater chance of finding approaches that work for them.

And remember how I mentioned that medicine's approach to mental health is constantly updated, as new information and understanding are taken into account? Much of that new info comes from the research conducted by psychologists. And, these days, neuroscientists.† Having said all that, there are still times when psychiatrists and psychologists butt heads.

Psychologists, particularly clinical ones, are a common feature of mental healthcare, regularly working alongside psychiatrists. They usually handle the more mild-to-moderate-

* Well, maybe you could? I doubt it would be a very successful one, though. But then, sport isn't my thing.
† No, honestly, don't mention it.

but-enduring cases, providing face-to-face talking therapies, like cognitive behavioural therapy, for patients who are willing and able to engage with such approaches. Or, they're dealing with a patient's long-term rehabilitation or care, where appropriate.

Some people scoff at talking therapies, but they're often very helpful, even for those who have their doubts, as Guy Kelly experienced . . .

I had cognitive behavioural therapy on the NHS and really recommend it. I know it's not right for everybody, but it worked for me. A thing I found useful about it particularly was just chatting with somebody who said 'How are you?', and meant it. I didn't have to follow up with, 'Oh, fine! How are you – how are things?' – it wasn't a superficial 'How are you?'. It was like, my job is literally to know how you are, so crack on, don't ask me about my day. You don't really get a chance to do that, normally.

It was really helpful, and great to see things written down. When you're trapped inside these things they can feel so big and so impossible to escape. But when you sit with somebody, with a pen and paper, and you write down your thought process like it's a flow chart for a company, it looks like this small, pitiful, pathetic thing that it is. It's like peering behind the curtain – something that you thought was huge and monstrous is reduced to just a few lines. And it felt like something that had previously had me trapped; I'd managed to trap it myself, like turning a glass on top of a particularly vicious spider.

Before I had CBT, my primary thought was, 'Well, I did a psychology A level, I'm just gonna know all the things they're looking for and give the answers they want to hear.' But obviously that's bullshit because it's their job; these people are trained for this, and they're specifically trained to deal with wankers like me who think they're smarter than the person they're talking to.

Mental healthcare is often provided by multidisciplinary teams, and this is very helpful. Mental disorders and the like have so many factors and manifestations that you *should* have many different experts addressing them.

Sadly, basic human nature means that such arrangements will often lead to group rivalries and spats, particularly when one side is higher in the pecking order than others. In this context, it's invariably psychiatrists who wield the most power (on paper, at least). This isn't exclusive to mental healthcare, of course; if you've ever had a baby in the UK's NHS and seen the deep suspicion some midwives have for doctors, you know what I'm getting at.

But it's not just turf wars or workplace politics. The psychiatrist-and-psychologist conflict, where it exists, does have some theoretical, even ideological basis. My own take is that it's often down to them approaching the same problem from opposite directions. Psychiatry tries to incorporate problems with the human mind into established systems of medicine, i.e. 'This is how medicine works, how do we apply this to mental health?' Psychologists, alternatively, try to incorporate medical and therapeutic approaches into the established understanding of the mind, i.e. 'This is how the mind works, what can we do to fix it if it goes wrong?'

If the medical model is flawed, the work of psychologists has, helpfully, provided several other approaches for addressing poor mental health. The most familiar is probably the cognitive model.[18] This underpins cognitive behavioural therapy, the most common talking therapy you hear about today, as well as many other similar techniques, like group therapies, family therapy, self-directed counselling, and so on.

While diagnosis is useful for medical interventions, it's not as much of a priority for clinical psychological approaches. Some psychoanalytical methods, another type of approach, argue that diagnosis is of no use,[19] because each individual patient is different enough to warrant a unique therapeutic approach tailored to their needs. It's as if every unwell person gets a disease named after them.

Cognitive models and psychoanalytic models have a lot of similarities, but also some key differences.[20] Cognitive models work towards helping individuals consciously learn to think in different, less debilitating ways; to sort of work through, or around, the mental issues they're experiencing. Psychoanalytic approaches, by contrast, are more focused on finding the cause, the particular event or trauma or aspect of your life that led to the current problems, usually via the effects experienced at unconscious levels.

These are just two well-known psychological methods with different approaches. But as mentioned, one thing they have in common is a focus on the patient and their specific expression of poor mental health, rather than adhering to a specific and familiar diagnosis.

A clinical psychologist I spoke to backed this up, likening their role to a chef who has to prepare specific recipes based on what ingredients the patient presents them with, rather than picking the recipe and trying to find what ingredients you need. The latter approach risks leaving things out, or making substitutions, which could end up ruining the recipe.

Broadly speaking, this method argues that, when it comes to mental disorders, it's not the underlying problems and causes that should be dealt with, but how the patient *thinks and feels* about them. If a certain life event, like losing your job, leaves you feeling hopeless and despairing, this shows a problem with cognition – with how you perceive and process the event – and it's this cognitive response that needs to be changed.

Take phobias, for example. If you've got arachnophobia, you're irrationally afraid of spiders. But it's your *response* to them that is the problem, not the spiders. They're not doing anything wrong, they're just existing.* Addressing the unhelpful response, the disruptive thought processes, is the goal of the cognitive model.

Let's try another analogy. Imagine your usual route home involves crossing a bridge over a river. One day, the bridge collapses while you're on the wrong side. You can't go home now, you're stuck. In this analogy, your house is your normal functioning mind. The bridge is your usual way of achieving

---

* Which is bad enough for some people, admittedly.

and sustaining it. The collapse is a traumatic life event, or whatever it is, that causes your mental health to suffer. What do you do about this situation, where you can't get to your 'normal' state?

If you adopt the medical model approach, that would involve someone coming along and trying to repair the bridge, or set up some other way of crossing, like a zipline or pontoon arrangement. They may not have the right tools for the job in hand, their alternatives may be riskier than the previous methods, and there's much trial and error involved. They may not even succeed in the end, but at least they're having a go, and it's often the fastest approach if you need to get home soon. But you mostly have to sit there and let them get on with it, no matter how cold and wet you are.

Alternatively, say someone appears and, rather than trying to fix the bridge, offers to help you find an alternative route across the river. They don't know the area, but they've got a compass and some spare boots, and offer to wander with you upstream, drawing a map as you go, until you find a new way home. In this example, that second person is using the cognitive model. The problem is still there, the bridge is still collapsed, but your response to it has changed; with help from someone else, you've found a new way of achieving normal functioning by incorporating and working around the existing problem.

This is what's deemed a top-down approach. Rather than fixing the underlying problem and letting everything hopefully click back into place, you figure out how to ignore or avoid the problem, thus nullifying its effects. For someone

67

with depression, for example, you wouldn't try to restore faulty levels of neurotransmitters or anything like that. You'd instead focus on preventing the types of thinking that sustain depression; inferring negative meanings to harmless conversation, exaggerated self-criticism, magnifying unpleasant outcomes and minimising good ones. All of these are modes and habits of thinking that can, with effort, be changed. Obviously, this approach has limits; for instance, it requires weeks of careful discussion and analysis, something invariably beyond those enduring a serious mental episode. But you can hopefully see how it appeals to many.

Of course, as is usually the case with anything regarding mental health, CBT has its criticisms and detractors. I've spoken to many individuals with chronic mental health issues who find the whole approach somewhat demeaning, insulting even, because it often boils down to someone telling you *how to feel*, or telling you what your problems are, and how to fix or avoid them. No matter how well trained or experienced they may be, having someone else lecture you about what's happening *in your own head* is a tricky thing for many to simply accept.

There's also the concern that, in stark contrast to the medical model, CBT and talking therapies put *too much* onus on the individual. As we'll soon see, many mental health problems have valid external causes; something negative has happened – or continues to happen – in someone's life, which undermines their mental health in debilitating ways. Teaching someone to think differently about a valid problem arguably doesn't 'deal with it', it just masks the symptoms.

And for many, that's not much different to being told to 'cheer up' or 'stay positive' when you've legitimate reasons to be unhappy. The medical model may have its many flaws, but at least it involves tangible efforts to deal with actual problems, so some still prefer this approach over the more cognitive one.

Thankfully, these different approaches aren't mutually exclusive. A combined approach, involving, for example, medication, counselling and cognitive therapies, can be most effective.[21] Many report that antidepressants helped them regain enough functioning to engage in cognitive talking therapy. Why not have someone fixing the bridge while you look for a new way around? There are other psychological models and methods of using them to tackle mental health problems, but, as mentioned earlier, a lot of the time they're handled by multidisciplinary teams, where different people with different expertise provide help where needed to tackle relevant facets of the patient's condition.

While psychiatrists and psychologists regularly combine their efforts, it's worth pointing out that there are those in psychology and related fields who dispute the whole principle of the medical, psychiatric approach to mental disorders altogether. For instance, in 2018 the esteemed BBC ran an article on their website titled 'Mental health is a myth', all about the new anti-psychiatry scholarship launched by the University of Toronto's Dr Bonnie Burstow,[22] an experienced psychotherapist.*

---

* Dr Burstow sadly passed away in January 2020.

Isn't it a bit . . . weird? A trained psychotherapist, insisting there's no such thing as mental health? Isn't that like a famous jockey denying the existence of horses? But clearly there are many out there who agree with this position. At least enough to warrant a scholarship, apparently. Why? How?

Based on my own understanding – which could easily be wrong, admittedly – while there are myriad reasons for people being opposed to the system and process of psychiatry, it seems many psychologists reject the whole notion of diagnosing people with mental disorders from the get-go. The rationale is that if you attach a label to someone stating they have a medical problem, that itself is a potentially harmful act.

You can't measure someone's mental state against robust and reliable baselines, and many argue that you shouldn't even try, because you could well be wrong and cause someone to undergo therapies and interventions that are harmful. We've seen how important the right language is in mental health, and the act of diagnosis, by definition, tells both the individual and the wider world that there's something *wrong*.

Numerous psychologists argue that this is not the case. Ever. There is, in fairness, a certain logic to refuting the very concept of mental disorders, or illnesses, one that sometimes crosses over into the philosophical.

Everything we perceive and comprehend is derived from crude raw data from our senses, having undergone extensive polishing, interpretation and extrapolation by our brains, right? So, who's to say that things like hallucinations and delusions seen in psychosis are any less valid an interpretation of the world than more typical perception? Indeed, many scientists and psychiatrists now acknowledge that practically everyone experiences hallucinations and delusions on a regular basis,[23] like religious experiences, ghostly encounters, conspiracy theories, and so on. It's said to be due to the way our brains try to impose some sort of structure on an increasingly complex and uncertain world. But the main point is, if we're all on some form of 'hallucinatory spectrum', why should people on the further ends be singled out as flawed?

Similarly, it could be argued that things like anxiety and depression are logical and normal, even *healthy* reactions to traumatic events or an increasingly stressful and complicated world; something we humans, and particularly our brains, haven't evolved to handle. Overall, a lot of the anti-psychiatry, anti-mental-illness arguments boil down to the stance that it's the society around us – our expectations and norms – that is too rigid and restrictive. It doesn't accommodate these alternative ways of thinking and being, so we class them as disordered and unwell, when we shouldn't.

Therefore, the real way to solve mental health 'issues' is for our overall understanding to change and adapt, to incorporate and accommodate those who don't conform to the narrowly defined norms. This can be achieved by changes in language, changes in definitions, changes in existing models, and, logically, by not assuming that anyone who doesn't conform to rigid norms has a medical problem that needs fixing, which is what diagnosis and the medical system does by definition. Even the term 'mental health' is suspect from this point of view. The very notion of health suggests something that can be poor or go wrong.

As I said, this is just my personal understanding of the logic behind some of the more vehement anti-psychiatry arguments, not including the ideological, political, or cult- or conspiracy-led ones. Apologies to anyone I've misrepresented here.

However, in the interest of balance, given how I highlighted the problems with the medical model at length, there are many flaws with psychological approaches too. There's a lot less consensus in the field of psychology overall than there is in medicine. While the medical consensus is largely written down in the DSM and ICD, the psychological approaches are a lot more varied. You get your Jungians and Freudians, your behaviourists, your existentialists, your developmental psychologists, your Gestalt psychologists, and so on. Last I checked, the list of known psychological approaches on Wikipedia is forty-five entries long. Which is a lot.

In fairness, rather than rival approaches, many of these can instead be likened to doctors specialising in different areas of medicine; they're just focusing on different aspects of the broader whole that is the mind. And most psychologists acknowledge the valid aspects of each different branch of the discipline, adopting more of an eclectic evidence-based approach.

But it's hard to build a concrete consensus when dealing with something as chaotic as the human mind and brain. And when different theories and perspectives are jostling for dominance in a limited pool of resources and funding, there are many times when ideologies can become the driving force behind behaviour. Sad as it may be, thanks to the wonders of social media I've seen psychologists who are flat-out opposed to psychiatry, or more mistrustful or resentful of it and its methods, angrily challenging or attacking individuals who speak out in favour of it. Such individuals are often actual mental health patients and activists, who have bravely opened up about their own serious issues. The last thing they need, or deserve, is clinical professionals criticising or condemning their own life experiences, or even telling them they're wrong when they say they're unwell. This is in no way a helpful approach, and not something I'd ever personally condone.

So, taking all this into account, what's *my* overall view? And where does all this leave those who struggle with their mental health and want something done about it?

The current understanding of mental health overall

What have we learned here? It may have seemed excruciatingly detailed, but what I've covered is mostly a whistle-stop tour of just some of the more fundamental properties and debates occurring in the world of mental health today.

Going back to the mental-health-as-a-festival analogy, I've just shown you the map of the site and pointed out the main locations. But to truly understand and appreciate how it all operates, and to find your way to where you want to go, you need to get in there and do some wandering around, which is what I'm hoping to do in the following chapters.

But before I do that, let's just remind ourselves of a few of the important points.

Firstly, while I try to avoid using the term mental illness if possible, I've no particular beef with anyone who does. I stick to 'disorder' or 'problem' where I can. But this doesn't mean I agree with the more extreme view that mental health *can't* go wrong. I've seen too many people I care about enduring deep discomfort and pain, thanks to their minds or brains turning against them, to accept that poor mental health isn't a thing. Such approaches, in my experience, readily lead to dismissing and ignoring people's genuine problems.

Also, and perhaps more relevantly to me and my expertise, it implies that the human brain *cannot* go wrong. Trust me, it definitely can. If you spend any length of time studying it, that becomes very clear, very quickly. So, I say that mental disorders and other problems *are* real; they have legitimate causes, they do need addressing, and any valid option that could provide help or solutions should be considered. That's the approach I'll be using in the next chapters. If you have any strong objections to any of that, we're going to have to agree to disagree.

And is there a particular model I use when approaching mental health? Cognitive, medical, psychoanalytical, or something else? Technically, since I don't do anything with patients, I don't need to stick to a specific approach. If you're just talking about mental health in the abstract, you can refer to all of them if you like. However, with that in mind, I tend to defer to the biopsychosocial model of mental health. It's what I was taught about, it's what I taught others about, and it's one of the more common approaches used today.[24]

As the name suggests, it acknowledges the complex, multifaceted nature of mental health, and the many different

74

factors that can disrupt it. Our physical body can be affected by physical things, like infection and injury. But, as we've seen, our minds are more intangible, so can be negatively affected by physical things *and* patterns of thought *and* external experiences. Properly understanding and handling mental health problems will involve all these factors, to a greater or lesser extent.

The biopsychosocial model is a means of considering them all, and asserts that mental health can be affected by three different levels of causes.

There's the biological level, including such things as genetic influences, chemical imbalances, drugs, toxins, and so on.

Then there's the psychological level, including unhelpful forms of thinking and cognition, sustained bad moods, reluctance to do things that improve health, etc.

Finally, there's the social level, covering traumatic events, bad relationships, an impoverished and stressful living environment, and so on.

These all feed into and influence each other. If a chemical imbalance causes you to become depressed, you experience a change in your thinking, and become trapped in a low-mood, zero-motivation state. This then means you can't work or socialise, so your employers and friends start treating you differently. This causes further stress via the social level, which impacts on our biological health, and the whole cycle starts all over again.

The biopsychosocial model was first proposed by George Engel way back in 1977, and eventually became the default approach of much of mental healthcare the world over. As a model, it was devised to counter the narrow focus and bio-logical or pharmacological biases of the more dogmatically medical approaches. But at the same time, it was intended to provide a more rational, scientific framework than the more individualistic mental health methods practised at the time, where each practitioner could arguably do their own thing.

The biopsychosocial model technically adds structure and reliability, while encompassing all possible aspects that can lead to health problems, essentially leaving no stone unturned. It's often used by psychiatrists when trying to determine exactly what is wrong with a patient, and what is the best way to manage it.

For instance, if a patient presents with memory problems, you don't just try and figure out what's going amiss with their brain, you take their whole situation into account. How old are they? Do they drink or take any medication? Any previous health problems? And when treating the issue, you don't just hand them some pills and boot them out, you see if they live alone, or have family, or are in an isolated area, or somewhere where they may be more prone to injuries, or have access to care in the community, and so on.

Of course, when it comes to actually assessing and treating patients, every approach covered so far has numerous limita-tions and criticisms. The medical model can focus too much on dealing with underlying biological issues. The cognitive model is a lengthy and elaborate approach, one that some-times ignores the cause while putting too much pressure on the patient. The quantitative approach used by abnormal psychology requires measuring and evaluating psychological traits, which is a very big ask.

And of course, the biopsychosocial model has problems too. Such as, where does one 'level' end and another begin? At what point does a biological problem become a psychological one? Is separating them in the first place all that wise? We've seen how medical science regularly needs certainty and clear definitions, and the biopsychosocial model often makes this harder, not easier.

There are also those who argue that this approach is essentially saying that *every* facet is equally important. In practical terms, this can be the same as saying *none* is most important: the everyone's-a-winner method, but in a mental health context. It can render the whole concept of having a rigorous, evidence-based approach meaningless. There are just so many factors to take into account, and addressing them all is seriously impractical, so the clinician can end up just going with what they deem the best course of action. This is an approach the biopsychosocial model was *devised to prevent*. It's also a pretty big ask to expect any individual to learn every single biological, psychological and social element of a patient's life.

All these things are true, and it's an ongoing debate and discussion, or argument, in the psychiatric and clinical psychology communities, as to which approach or model is best. Lucky for me, it's not my job to actually treat patients, so I tend to use the biopsychosocial approach as more of a 'jumping-off' point. It helps to stay alert to the fact that mental health problems are the product of all these different factors, and I'll do my best to consider all of them in the coming chapters.

Given all I've covered regarding the current state of mental healthcare in the modern world, you'd be forgiven for thinking it seems like something of a confusing mess. Maybe that's appropriate, what with how complicated and baffling mental health itself is. Fight fire with fire, and all that.

But still, there are so many approaches and ideologies and schools of thought, all derived from a constantly changing evidence base, and judged against ever-shifting social norms. Considering all that, the obvious question is: how does anything get done at all? Can we trust *anything* told to us about mental health, by those charged with addressing it when it goes wrong?

I'd say yes, of course we can.

There's a famous saying: A camel is a horse designed by a committee. It's usually used to emphasise that the more people involved in a process, the more convoluted and inefficient the outcome. In this context, a complete and perfect understanding of mental health, and what to do when it goes wrong, is a horse. Therefore, our current approach to mental health problems, and how to deal with them, is the proverbial camel, produced by a horse-designing committee. With so many different contributions and approaches and theories and ideas from an ever-changing understanding of what is and isn't 'normal', it was never going to be sleek and simple.

However, in this instance, that's not exactly a bad thing. When you consider that nobody involved knows what a horse looks like, a camel is actually a pretty good result. If what you need is a horse but what you've got is a camel, it's not a total disaster. It might not be as efficient or obedient, but you can still make progress, and get things done.

My point is, the modern-day approach to, and understanding of, mental health may be imperfect, but it's certainly better than nothing. And it's the result of an immeasurable amount of time, effort and energy from literally millions of well-informed, intelligent people. It can still be, and regularly is, extremely helpful, and saves countless lives.

Overall, there's still a great deal we don't know about mental health. But there's also a great deal we *do* know. And that knowledge is used in a wide variety of ways.

That's what this book is about. It's an attempt to reveal to the everyday person our modern understanding of mental health, and how this is used to deal with the issues surrounding it. And, to bring it full circle, pretty much all of it can be brought back to the workings of the brain. There are times when the brain just goes wrong, and our mental health suffers.

There are also times when our brain isn't going wrong per se, but it's ended up doing wrong or unhelpful things, so our mental health suffers. It's sort of like when a computer gets a virus; there's a problem that needs addressing, but you don't need to replace the processor or motherboard. It's functioning fine, it's just being made to do something unhelpful.

Also, everyone's brain is different. The way brains form is based on countless different factors, from DNA to hormones to experiences to diet to the environment, and more. So, while people's brains may look the same from the outside, at the deeper microscopic levels, the specific arrangements of

79

connections between the billions of cells that make up your brain – connections that determine who you are and how you function – are unique to you, more than any fingerprint could ever be.

So, some drugs will work on some people, and make things worse for others. Some people will respond well to cognitive talking therapies, others won't. Certain people will experience the exact same underlying problem in wildly different ways to others.

And because it's not a simple logic machine, there are countless tics and impulses and biases and imbalances in the human brain that affect how we experience, observe and respond to mental health, and the problems that can occur with it.

It's my intention to explore all of this and how it applies to specific disorders in the following chapters. Specifically, the most common mental health disorders seen in the wider world today. These tend to be of the neurotic variety: the mood or anxiety disorders. While psychotic disorders, eating disorders and personality disorders are widespread and definitely require more attention and understanding, it's impossible for anyone to cover *every* aspect of mental health problems in one single book.

In my defence, even focusing on the more common disorders and attempting to explain them is a very big task; one there's a good chance I'll fail at.

But at least I tried. And that's the main thing, right?

2: How the brain works

So, what's happening in the brain when we experience mental health issues?

Well, before I can answer that, I feel I need to make sure everyone is aware of the basics. It's not much use explaining what happens when the brain goes wrong if we don't actually know what's happening when it's going *right*. Because there's no point in giving a detailed explanation of the neuroscience underlying mental health matters if the person hearing it has no idea what I'm talking about. You might as well just spend ten minutes making fart noises with your armpits. They'll be no less enlightened, and at least they might get a giggle out of that.

But it's very useful to know the fundamentals of the brain if you're going to apply neurological processes to matters as tricky as mental health. It's like how you need to have a good grasp of human anatomy if you want to be a medic, particularly if you want to be a surgeon. If there's one thing you don't want to hear from a surgeon, as you go under, it's 'What the hell is *that*?'*

Basically, a general understanding of the key properties of the brain may prove vital for your understanding of the

* For any *Simpsons* fans, yes, that is what Homer hears his surgeon, Doctor Nick Riviera, say as the anaesthetic kicks in for his heart bypass, in one of my favourite jokes from the show.

disorders and problems I'll be covering in the rest of this book.

So, let's address the structure and workings of the brain. We'll be looking at the most fundamental building blocks, the genes and molecules that make up brain cells and provide their special, vital properties. We'll be looking at how these brain cells communicate, by passing signals back and forth, which is what allows us to have a mind go awry. And we'll explore the structure and layout of the brain, the clusters and networks and circuits, the things that give rise to such complexity and rich detail when it comes to what goes on in our heads.

The most basic elements of brain activity

Like pretty much everything else in your body, the brain is made of cells. So far, so good.

Usually, when people refer to brain cells, they mean *neurons*. You've probably seen images of them. They're those vaguely spiky, branching cells that look a bit like a cross between a tree and a spider. However, while many people refer to neurons as brain cells, that's not strictly accurate, as they aren't found solely in the brain. They make up your whole nervous system, like your spinal cord, and all the nerves spread throughout your body, regulating and controlling your physiological systems, feeding back information from your senses and peripherals, and so on.

Also, it's not *just* neurons that make up the brain and nervous system. There are other kinds of cells in there, often labelled glia, or support cells. These cells essentially keep the brain together, in one piece. They support, protect, assist and maintain neurons. They're like the entourage – the minders and bodyguards and personal assistants – for neurons, which are the performers.* These support cells are as numerous as neurons in the brain, and just as crucial: we wouldn't survive a second without them. However, I'm going to put them aside and just concentrate on neurons, because those are the ones that do all the things this book focuses on. If I say 'brain cells' from this point on, I mean neurons.

Neurons usually have one big central mass, or hub, called a cell body. They have lots of little limbs or branches, known as dendrites, and they usually have one big trunk-type appendage called an axon. These can be pretty long, with the longest being the sciatic nerve,[1] running from your spine to the end of your leg, over a metre in length. That might not sound like much, but when we're talking about a single cell, it's a ludicrous distance. And nerves, those long, stringy, squishy cables that run everywhere through our bodies? These are essentially bundles of neurons, woven together like the individual threads that make up a thick rope.

There are around a hundred billion neurons in the brain, and practically everything the brain does, from basic functions like controlling breathing or movement to frightfully complex actions like language processing and imagination, is based on energetic activity in neurons. Or, perhaps more accurately, energetic activity *between* neurons. So, let's look

---

* Or, in some cases, divas.

at what this activity actually is, and how it works. Because we'd literally be nothing without it.

Firstly, all cells have what's called a membrane potential. The membrane is the skin of the cell, a layer of fatty molecules that keeps the *inside* of the cell separate from the *outside* of the cell. Sounds simple, but when at the molecular scale, such distinctions aren't as clear-cut as you might hope, so this is very important.

Then we have the cellular medium. It's basically the substance in which cells reside, or live, or sit, or whatever. For fish in the ocean, seawater is their medium. For us humans, oxygen-infused air is our medium. For your cells, it's a sort of molecularly enriched liquid, which takes various forms throughout our bodies and tissues.

This cellular medium is, in most large creatures,* labelled the extracellular fluid. It's basically a way of describing all the fluid inside your body that *isn't* inside a cell. Makes sense. The fluid that specifically surrounds and supports cells is called interstitial fluid. But never mind the name right now, just focus on the fact that it's vital for keeping us alive.

This might sound excessive, because how can a bit of nondescript liquid, not even good enough to enter the cells, be so important? Well, we're mammals, meaning we've evolved to control and regulate many of our internal life-sustaining processes, like our body temperature. These are all regulated largely at the cellular level by sophisticated, delicate, and mind-numbingly complex exchanges of chemicals. And the

* Meaning, any creature we can see without a microscope.

84

interstitial fluid contains all these chemicals, and allows them to move around. To say that interstitial fluid is important for keeping us alive is like saying the planet Earth is important for keeping cities in place.

So, the interstitial fluid is a complex broth of crucial chemicals. And it's chock-full of ions,* which, in this case, are *positively charged* atoms and molecules. However, the cell membrane, the complex layer of lipids and fats that forms the 'skin' of the cell, keeps most of these ions out. The result here is that there are more positively charged ions *outside* the cell than *inside*.

If it helps, think of the cell as a bouncy castle at a fete, and the ions are kids that want to play on it. But they can't all go on it at once; that would cause damage and injuries, and make the whole set-up unworkable. So, stewards at the bouncy castle entrance (i.e. the cell membrane) only allow a certain number of children in and out. This would inevitably end up with far more children outside the bouncy castle waiting to get in than children inside the bouncy castle trying to get out. So, you get more ions outside the cell than in.

But the key detail is that the ions carry a small positive electrical charge. And if there's more of them outside than inside, there's a higher level of positive charge on the outside of the cell membrane than on the inside, because there are more ions out there. This difference in charge sets up an electrical potential, a voltage, at the cell's surface, also known as a resting membrane potential.[2]

* Why? Well . . . because chemistry, that's why.

The specifics of electrical activity and how it works are best left to physicists to explain, but to put it simply, the surface of all cells is electrically active. There's a chemically induced voltage there, just like in a battery – albeit a very small one, given how cells are microscopic.

You might think . . . so what? Cells are slightly electrically active, but so are balloons if you rub them enough. What does it matter? Well, again, without this resting membrane potential, life as we know it *could not exist*. Cells wouldn't be able to do anything useful. It's admittedly a tricky concept, but it's very relevant. Because while this vital resting membrane potential, this imbalance in electrical charge, is present in all cells, neurons are special, because they can *change* it.

Neurons can, when circumstances require, alter the way a certain part of their membrane works. Specialised molecules in the membrane act as channels and gates and pumps for ions, and can be activated in particular circumstances, meaning positive ions *can* flood through the membrane, with the result that the inside becomes *more* positive than the outside. This sets up a different voltage compared to the usual resting potential. It goes from around *minus* seventy millivolts to *plus* forty millivolts. Again, might not sound like much, but it's a *huge* deal.

The thing is, this typically only happens at one small part of the neuron's membrane surface. But because of the way electrical charges and fluid environments and chemical gradients work, and the fact that there's nothing separating this point of electrical change from the more typical fluid around it, this change in membrane voltage spreads, out and away from the point where it occurred, and travels along the membrane of the neuron.

A simpler way of thinking of it is that it's like dropping a pebble into a still pond. The ripples travel outwards along the water's surface, from the point where the pebble broke the surface, right? But the water hasn't changed, nor has the air above its surface. The ripple isn't really a single separate 'thing', but it's still definitely there. It's a travelling point of *change*. This change in the electrical properties of the neuron membrane is a lot like that; it's a ripple, a localised but moving change, in the otherwise consistent boundary between two mediums. Except, rather than air and water, it's an electrical – or electrochemical, if you prefer – change, travelling along the membrane of neurons, between two microscopic fluid environments.

However, this ripples-in-the-water comparison only goes so far, because the water in a pond is essentially passive in the whole process; it's not really doing anything to help the ripples along. But imagine if it were. Imagine if the water could somehow deliberately shape, direct, even accelerate the ripples that occur when a pebble is dropped into it.

If it were possible to direct and focus the ripples, so they only go where you want them to go rather than spread out everywhere, you could send them to specific locations. If you could create new ripples quickly and in rapid succession, you could form complex messages, like some sort of Morse code. Two ripples for yes, three for no, four for the letter A, and so on. And if you could somehow accelerate the ripples, you could send them along at a much higher speed. Putting all

87

this together, you could use this surreal pond to send complex information, very quickly, to specific locations, via the ripples in its surface.

Bizarre as it sounds, this hypothetical 'smart pond' is essentially what the membrane of a neuron is like. It's studded with complex specialised molecules that allow the 'action potential' – this change in electrical imbalance that exists in all cells – to occur, before returning it to normal. Not only that, they help *direct* the action potential, channelling it from one end of the neuron to the other. They can even accelerate it.

Why? What's all this for? Well, those signals, those microscopic bursts of electrical activity occurring in neurons known as action potentials,[3] are what your brain uses to do . . . pretty much everything. There are immeasurable trillions of them happening throughout your brain and nervous system, for every second of your existence. Every thought, every movement, every sensory experience you have: all are the end result of action potentials, occurring in certain parts of the brain and nervous system. They are the signals that pass from neuron to neuron, that allow the brain to do all the complex processes and calculations it needs to do. They are to your mind, your consciousness, what atoms are to a tree, what words are to a novelist – simple things in isolation, but which can be combined and expressed in ways that end up being unbelievably rich and complex.

Here's why I tell you all this. Firstly, with this information, you can hopefully begin to see how the brain, that ugly lump of fat and grease housed in our skulls, can give rise to thoughts and language and motivations and emotions and experiences, and so on. Secondly, and more specifically, these action potentials, and all that they do, can only happen because of the very unique and specific structure and properties of neurons. The structure of neurons is, thanks to the dictates of nature and chemistry, determined by the molecules they're made up of. And these molecules? A lot of them are proteins.

Proteins play countless vital roles in the structure and functioning of a cell. In this case, remember those sophisticated molecules in the neuron's membranes, those gates and channels that allow action potentials to occur and be used in such sophisticated ways? Those are proteins. And proteins are what genes – dedicated sections of our DNA – produce. That's basically what DNA is *for*: it's a mammoth set of instructions for assembling every protein needed to make an organism. In this case, us. DNA does other stuff too, but that's the main thing (as far as we know).

And if DNA is a set of instructions for making the proteins that we need for us to exist, it's undeniably *very* important that these instructions are correct. Proteins are long chains of amino acids (a smaller, less complex type of molecule) folded up in very complicated three-dimensional ways, like a sort of microscopic origami where you can fold the paper several thousand times. The eventual shape of the protein is crucial in allowing it to do what it needs to do, and the shape is determined by the precise sequence of the chain of molecules it's assembled from. And if this sequence is not one hundred per cent correct, the shape of the protein changes, and it may

89

well not be able to do its job properly – if at all. And given the function of DNA, that's essentially what genetic problems, unhelpful changes in someone's DNA, do: introduce errors into the structure of proteins.

If it helps, you can think of it like the instructions for building a Lego model. Each individual brick you add seems inconsequential by itself, but if you do it slightly wrong, introducing minor errors, this can cause disproportionately large disruptions to the process, meaning the eventual model is asymmetrical, or insufficiently sturdy, or can't form at all. Similarly, even a few amino acids out of place in the sequence can cause a lot of problems for a protein.

Much of the time, it's no big deal. DNA codes for *a lot* of proteins, and not all of them are completely vital. But if the affected protein is a key element of an important cellular process, one that our health depends upon, then it's a big problem.

For example, if a protein involved in the sending of action potentials is misshapen, then the neurons will be less capable of sending and regulating them. And a protein will be misshapen if the gene that contains the instructions for assembling it is wrong in some way. Remember, every cell in the body uses the same DNA, so if a protein is wrong in *one* cell, there's a good chance it'll be wrong in *all* of them.

And this is how mental health issues can, and do, have a genetic component. You can have a faulty gene that codes for a protein that has important roles in certain neurons. And these neurons may be a key element in a specific brain function. Therefore, the faulty gene means the functioning of those neurons is going to be compromised. And, logically, so is your brain's ability to perform whatever function those neurons are involved in. And if that role is an important part of maintaining your mental health? Well . . .

There are known to be genetic factors involved in a wide range of mental health issues.[4] Depression, anxiety, psychosis, addiction, schizophrenia, bipolar disorder; there's ample evidence all these and more have at least some genetic factors at work, which gives rise to heritability. As in, if one of your parents, or another family member, has a certain disorder, the odds of you developing the same disorder are somewhat higher than for someone very similar to you but with no family history of it. To put it as simply as possible, you and your family members have a lot of genes, a lot of DNA, in common, and if there's an issue with a relative's DNA that leads to a mental health problem, it's more likely that the same issue is present in your DNA.

It's not a straightforward yes-or-no thing, thankfully. There is no one specific gene that causes, for instance, depression, where you definitely won't get depression if that gene isn't part of your DNA, but you definitely will if it is. The brain is invariably too complex and convoluted to allow for such a simple set-up. Genetic factors in mental health problems are far more subtle, nudging development and functioning in unhelpful directions, but certainly not being the sole cause of problems. In many cases, we don't even know what the troublesome genes are; we can only infer their existence by looking at the data, seeing how often problems occur in specific family lines, and so on.

However, this isn't always the case. Sometimes, genetic factors are far more blatant in their effects. The most obvious example is Huntington's disease, which we know is caused by a specific gene, for the protein huntingtin.[5] In certain people, the chain of molecules that leads to the protein huntingtin is too long, due to some unfortunate glitch of genetics. Part of it repeats more than it should. It's as if, instead of 'huntingtin', their gene says 'huntingtintintintintintintintin'.

The exact function of this protein is presently unknown, but we know it's important for various aspects of the brain's structure and functioning, as the most classic symptoms of Huntington's disease are inability to control movements, and mood disorders. And degradation of several important brain regions. All this, because one part of the affected gene is longer than it should be, resulting in misshapen proteins.

Unfortunately, genetic factors in mental health problems are rarely as clear-cut as this, because the brain is so incredibly versatile, complex and adaptable. Also, the functioning and structure of your brain has as much to do with how you grow and develop as it does with what's in your DNA. The typical brain has a lot of redundancy too; it's always developing workarounds or alternative ways to do something if there's difficulty or disruption.

But still, its ability to do all this is finite. And if there's a genetic factor causing problems deep in the cellular processes that the brain relies on, this can often make the difference between an ability or an inability to deal with things that harm your mental health.

To summarise: your brain is made of neurons, aka brain

cells. And these neurons have special properties that allow them to create and send action potentials – signals – back and forth. These are what the brain uses to do literally everything, including when it comes to our minds: our thoughts, emotions, perception, and all that. But all this depends on the specific structure and make-up of neurons. And sometimes, misbehaving genes can introduce flaws and errors. So even at this depth, mental health problems can occur.

Now, here's the alarming bit. Despite how complicated this all sounds, it's still pretty much the *simplest* aspect of how the brain works. Your average brain takes these fundamental processes and builds even greater layers of complexity out of them. And this all feeds into our mental health too.

Let's zoom out a bit, and try to look at some other key features.

Gap the mind: the crucial role of synapses

Our minds, every thought, every action, every sensation we experience, are the result of action potentials, tiny bursts of information, that occur in neurons. So far, so good. The main point of action potentials is that they allow signals to be passed along and between neurons, and this allows the brain to do what it does. Such signals can end up pretty much anywhere in the brain – they can be relayed to neurons nearby, or to those right on the other side of the brain, the cellular equivalent of a person phoning someone on the other side of the planet.

However, given how these neuronal signals are infinitesimally small, and the brain is pretty big in comparison, wouldn't this be a slow process? You'd think so, but these signals can travel along neurons at nearly *half the speed of sound*! One hundred and twenty metres a second. The typical brain is about fifteen centimetres long, so this means information moves around your brain and nervous system at ludicrous speed. Admittedly, it's not as fast as in the electrical circuits of machines and computers, which transmit information at a decent fraction of light speed. That's why these devices process information so much faster than us. But still, neurons certainly conduct information quickly enough for our needs.

So, billions upon trillions of microscopic signals being bounced around a bafflingly complex network of delicate cells: how does that coalesce into the rich, unified experience that is the human mind, human consciousness? Well, yes, that's the question, isn't it? If you know the answer, do let people know, they've been trying to work it out for centuries.

But, back to what we *do* know.

One key aspect, especially when it comes to understanding mental health issues, concerns how neurons send signals to each other. We've seen how action potentials work, but here's the thing; most neurons aren't directly connected. Where one neuron meets another, they *don't physically touch*. There's a gap between them, known as a synapse, and a lot of very important stuff happens here.*

Action potentials, those signals that allow the brain to do everything, *can't cross the synapse*. They exist in the

---

* Yes, it's weird to think that a gap, an absence of something, might be important, but that's the brain for you.

membrane, the skin, of the neuron. If we go back to the analogy of ripples in the surface of a pond, you can send messages across the pond, but you couldn't use directed ripples to send information to another pond. Because a ripple can't go where there's no water. Similarly, a gap between neurons means there's nowhere for an action potential to go, no membrane for it to travel along. You can't cross a bridge that isn't there.

This issue is resolved with neurotransmitters. When a signal reaches the terminus of one neuron, that neuron squirts packets of dedicated chemicals, neurotransmitters, into the synapse, the gap. The neuron on the other side of the gap has dedicated receptors, yet more proteins embedded in the membrane, which receive and recognise the chemical neurotransmitter that's just been released. Presence of a neurotransmitter initiates the processes that produce a new signal, a new action potential, which then travels along that neuron, to the next synapse, where the whole process is repeated.

You could say the neurotransmitters are like keys, and the receptors in the next neuron are like the locked doors that are opened by said keys. Unlocking the doors allows the message to continue. Or, maybe it's more like a relay race? Where runners pass a baton to the next one in line. Without the baton, the race cannot continue. Except, instead of just passing a baton, the next runner in line must make a new baton, and carry that to the next person, who then does the same. That's sort of how neurons pass messages between each other.

You might think this is an inefficient system. Having to create a whole new signal each time you get to the next cell?

Wouldn't it be a lot quicker to just link them up and allow the signals to pass directly?

If we were just talking about long chains of neurons passing signals from one end to the other, then yes, it would be. But neurons do so much more than that. Neurons form loops and tangles and branches and junctions and borders, and so on and so on. In some cases, a single neuron can receive signals from thousands of other neurons, and a single neuron can relay signals to thousands of others. And these arrangements are regularly changing, shifting, updating, as the brain learns and adapts. If neurons were all permanently attached to each other, this couldn't happen. Keeping some space between them allows flexibility, adaptability and versatility – vital properties for the working brain.

As well as that, neurotransmitters allow a much wider range of options than just passing on a basic signal. Neurons deploy a very wide range of different neurotransmitters. You've probably heard of them. Dopamine, oxytocin, serotonin, these are all neurotransmitters. And there are often several different receptors that respond to them, in different ways. Essentially, the chemical messenger and receptor system provides far more options for what to communicate to the next cell.

For instance, some neurotransmitters are excitatory, meaning they increase the amount of activity in the following neuron, creating new signals as we've seen, or maybe even *amplifying* the signal produced by that neuron, like someone turning up the volume on a stereo. Other neurotransmitters are inhibitory, meaning they reduce the activity in the neuron they interact with, cutting off or cancelling the signal, like someone turning the stereo down, or off altogether.

Indeed, neurons that specialise in these types of transmitter are often labelled excitatory or inhibitory neurons, because they respectively increase or decrease the actions of the neurons they link to. The flexible, neurotransmitter-dependent system used by neurons allows many parts of the brain to fulfil multiple functions – perform various roles. Action potentials alone, although simpler, faster and easier to create, don't allow for such versatility. The point is, neurotransmitters and synapses may introduce some delay into neuronal communication, but it's worth the cost as they mean the type of information that can be passed around the brain, from cell to cell, is substantially richer and more diverse.

It's also worth mentioning that using this chemical messaging approach means the brain and body are far more intertwined than many realise. Remember those receptors, molecules embedded in neurons in a synapse, that recognise and respond to specific chemical neurotransmitters? You can find them in countless other cells too, that make up other tissues and organs in the body. Except instead of neurotransmitters, which are chemical messengers released by a neuron nearby, many of these receptors in other organs are triggered by *hormones*, chemical messengers in the bloodstream, which travel all around the body and into every organ and tissue.

In a way, hormones are to neurotransmitters what a physical letter is to an email. An email may be faster and more direct, while a letter has to travel around the entire postal system. But it'll get there eventually. And while a letter may travel round a whole city in a postal van, there's only one address it will be delivered to.

Hormones are like that; they may travel around your whole body, but they'll only have an effect on cells with the appropriate receptor. As well as the nervous system, the hormone system, known scientifically as the endocrine system, is a means via which your body's systems are regulated, controlled and coordinated. And because both hormones and neurotransmitters are essentially chemical messengers that interact with specific receptors, there's a lot of overlap. Sometimes, certain chemicals can perform double duty, as neurotransmitters *and* hormones.

Oxytocin, for example. Often called the 'cuddle hormone' because of its role in human emotion and bonding, it's found in both the bloodstream and dedicated neurons in the brain, meaning it has many different effects, depending on where and how it's deployed. There are even parts of the brain dedicated to releasing hormones into your bloodstream as and when required. The hypothalamus, a deep and fundamental part of the brain, oversees the neuroendocrine system. In plain English, this is where dedicated neurons in the brain squirt hormones into your blood, to trigger useful responses in organs elsewhere in the body. Also, hormones released elsewhere in the body can have direct effects on the brain, which is still another organ at the end of the day, so it's a two-way system.

This set-up is important for mental health and our understanding of it, for several reasons. Firstly, as with genes, our brains and minds are supported by the actions of countless chemicals operating in specific ways at specific times. But this means that if something goes wrong with these chemicals, then problems occur. Many people have heard or even used the phrase 'chemical imbalance' when discussing the nature of mental health problems. While the reality is actually much more complex than that, it's true that too much or too little of a crucial chemical can have profound consequences and cause serious problems. We'll explore this much more in the following chapters.

Secondly, if the whole of your brain and body is co-ordinated and controlled by a system of chemical messages, would it be possible to, in a sense, hijack that? To introduce chemicals into the body from the outside that send a different message, telling your brain and body to do something other than what it's doing?

Yes, that's entirely possible. That's basically what most drugs are – chemicals that have something in common with, or some similar property to, a specific type of chemical messenger found in the body. This similarity means they're recognised by the receptors that respond to our natural chemical messengers. Therefore, drugs can and do affect what's going on in certain cells, by mimicking, blocking, or otherwise altering the effect of the chemical messengers those cells usually respond to. Turns out, the drugs *do* work, and this is how.

Psychoactive drugs, in particular those used to tackle mental health problems, usually work by mimicking the actions of neurotransmitters, or otherwise influencing their release and use in synapses. This is how they affect the brain specific-ally. Of course, thanks to the bafflingly intricate nature of the

99

brain's wiring, the role and effect of drugs gets very confusing, very quickly. For instance, a drug may cause a certain type of neuron to increase its activity, but if that neuron is an inhibitory neuron, this will mean neurons downstream aren't as active. So, a drug that increases activity in a neuron ends up *stopping* something from happening. Like I said, it's confusing.

Another important issue is that, thanks to how the brain and hormone system are so intertwined, if something goes awry in the brain, it can lead to physical symptoms. If you're constantly experiencing unpleasant, negative thoughts and issues, then your body can be directly affected, because your brain, responding to these negative signals, can end up pumping chemical messages into your bloodstream, causing your physical system to respond, often in unhelpful ways. In this case, a worried brain, plagued by unpleasant thoughts, would release stress hormones into your bloodstream, causing muscle tension, irritability, appetite changes, and so on.*

If you were still wondering how a mental health problem can have physical consequences, this is how. The chemical communication system that your brain and body use to do literally everything means that, despite many people's scepticism, mental health issues are quite capable of leading to tangible physical consequences and symptoms. They absolutely are not 'all in your head'.

So, to summarise: your neurons communicate with each other via neurotransmitters, dedicated chemicals that can cause a

---

* We'll see a lot more about this in later chapters.

range of diverse outcomes. There are lots of different types of neurotransmitters, which produce lots of different outcomes. You could think of the suite of neurotransmitters the brain has access to as colours in the palette of a talented artist. The colours available may seem pretty limited, just red, orange, green, etc. But an artist can blend and combine and mix them, to create a breathtaking range of hues and shades and gradients and images. And the brain does exactly that, except with neurotransmitters and mental processes, not colours and pictures.*

There's also much overlap between the neurotransmitter system, where neurons communicate with and control each other, and the hormone system, where chemicals in the bloodstream are used to influence and control our body's organs and tissues. Indeed, the brain and body are fundamentally linked via this system, which explains how and why mental health issues can often have physical symptoms. And, in many cases, vice versa.

And finally, the fact that we can introduce new chemicals into these systems, via digestion, inhalation, injection or other means, is what gives us drugs. Drugs can influence and alter what the body and brain are doing, by interfering or co-opting the receptors that neurotransmitters and hormones act on, sort of like someone discovering your password and accessing your computer, to change all your settings.

* Although some of those neurotransmitters are used by the brain to create our rich colour perception, which is where this analogy becomes rather circular.

But before we get carried away, this is by no means an automatically helpful thing to do. Chemical messengers, as a term, may sound straightforward, but it doesn't even begin to do justice to just how complicated things get at this cellular level. After all, we barely know how most of it operates, even after centuries of study.

That's why drugs must be extensively and carefully researched and tested, because it's impossible to work out exactly how and why they'll affect us without doing so. Introducing a new, untested drug into the human body and brain would be like randomly flicking switches and pushing buttons at the controls of a jumbo jet. One in mid-flight, full of passengers. Basically, to bring up the useful piloting analogy again, just because you have access to the cockpit, it doesn't mean you know how to fly the plane. And even with our most advanced biosciences, modern understanding is still largely at the stage of signing up for piloting lessons.

We've seen how neurons work, and how they communicate, and the results of this. Now let's zoom out again, and see what happens when you pack a hundred billion neurons together, and make a brain.

Nuclei, networks and circuits: the big bits of the brain

The brain is made up of neurons, but it's not just a big ball of cells, clumped together. There are also different types, different classes, of neurons, with different shapes, properties, structures, using different neurotransmitters, and so on. The type of neurons that link up, and the ways in which they connect to each other, can make all the difference. Certain parts of the brain have certain types of neurons, assembled into one specific area, or region, or *bit*. And these different bits do different things, introducing yet more complexity and diversity.

However, before I go further with that, there's one thing it's important to get straight. You've probably seen pop science news stories before now, talking about some study that shows a certain part of the brain is responsible for a particular function, usually thanks to experiments conducted using brain-scanning technology. I've personally seen stories about the part of the brain responsible for Facebook addiction, love of Apple products, political leaning, religious belief, and more.

There's this persistent, and neuroscientifically annoying, mainstream tendency to present the brain as 'modular', meaning that it's made up of many specific parts, and each part is responsible for a specific thing, and *just* that thing. This, logically, would mean that there's one specific part dedicated to every single thing the brain is capable of. So, if you like ice cream, there's supposedly a 'liking ice cream' centre of the brain. If you play football, there's a football centre of the brain. And so on. This is a huge oversimplification at best, and at worst a severe misrepresentation of how the brain operates.

It's not that it's one hundred per cent inaccurate, because there are indeed different parts of the brain that fulfil different, distinct roles. Specific parts of the brain have been shown to be responsible for memory processing and retrieval, language, vision, motor control, and so on. You can also assign functional roles to different *regions* of the brain. The frontal regions, right behind your eyes, are pretty much the driving seat, responsible for rational thought, planning, attention, decision-making and self-control. The upper-middle areas of the brain, the parietal lobes, handle language, movement control, sensory stuff, and so on. The middle, side-on regions, the temporal lobes, handle a lot of memory and information processing like that. The rear of the brain, the occipital lobe, handles most of the visual processing.*

You may be thinking, doesn't all that completely contradict everything he said just now? About the idea of specific brain regions having dedicated roles being basically wrong? I'd argue that no, it doesn't. Because all these things I just listed are fundamental processes and functions, not something as nebulous and abstract as political leanings. Most people would struggle to accurately define their political views beyond all doubt, narrowing them down to specific and recognisable labels. It's a bit much to expect a brain scanner to somehow achieve this.

And even at the most straightforward, fundamental levels, there's still much overlap and ambiguity. The hippocampus, for example, is well established as being responsible for the creation of detailed long-term memories. But it's also heavily involved in spatial navigation, the ability to find your way around your environment. Why would one brain bit be used

---

* Interesting aside: when you hit your head, the impact causes your brain to bounce around inside your skull. And when the back of your brain hits the solid bone of your skull, the blunt force triggers your visual system in confusing ways, hence you 'see stars' when you receive a blow to the head.

to perform two such distinct roles? Isn't that like trying to butter your toast with a calculator? Not really. Those might sound like very different things, but given how you need to have information about where you've been and where you're going in order to navigate efficiently, maybe memory and navigation are both supported by a system for storing information from the senses in practically useful ways.

That's one theory anyway. The point is, while certain parts of the brain are indeed specialised for specific fundamental processes, these processes are used in a variety of ways, so in most cases the different parts perform *multiple* functions. And from the outside, these functions look like a very mixed bag. Think of it like the alphabet. The alphabet, in English at least, is just twenty-six single letters. Doesn't sound like much. But these letters are used to create sentences, poems, essays, books, sonnets, songs, love letters, ransom demands, and so much more. It's all the same simple elements, being used and applied in a dizzying range of complex ways. This is something the brain does a lot.

And on top of that, even the most distinct parts of the brain are connected to almost every other region, either directly or indirectly, so everything can influence everything else, to a greater or lesser extent. If we stick with the alphabet example, you know how in certain words the arrangement of letters can influence how they're pronounced, or how they work? Like how P suddenly sounds like F when you put it in front of an H? The brain's a lot like that, except that in the brain's case, words at the very end of a paragraph, or even at the end of a novel, can affect how the ones at the *start* are pronounced.

It may sound a recipe for absolute chaos, and yes, a lot of the time it can be, but at the same time it's vitally important. It's another arrangement that gives the human brain so much power and diversity.

Indeed, while the more fundamental processes like senses and memory can be pinned to specific regions or bits of the brain, the more abstract, intangible things the human brain does are more often attributed to networks. They're produced via the activity of multiple different areas working together, giving rise to processes and abilities that are very different to what they'd be able to do alone.

Intelligence, for example. Despite efforts to find one, there's no decent evidence that there's one specific part of the brain that is responsible for intelligence. Indeed, many scientists still argue about what intelligence actually *is*. But however you'd define it, most data suggest intelligence is a product of many different brain regions, processing information in a diverse range of ways.

And that's where the clichéd 'a big brain means you're smarter' assumption comes undone. While it's something a lot of people think is true, it really isn't. Differences in intelligence don't seem to have any real link to differences in brain size, at least not when you're comparing humans to other humans.

While certain people are undoubtedly more intelligent than others, this is likely to be due to efficiency, as in how well and how easily the network of different brain regions responsible for intelligence work together, to fulfil their role. The better and more well-connected the brain network is, the more intelligent the person. Think of it as a team of people working together on a specific task, like designing a house. If they're working together in the same building, able to share ideas and plans and designs with ease, they'll get a lot more done in a shorter space of time. But if they were all working separately in different cities or different time zones, they'd have to rely on the mail system or phone network, contending with delays and technical limitations and confusion and uncertainty.

In the first scenario, the team can communicate very efficiently. In the second, not so much. The thing is, it's the same team in both cases, but the way in which they're connected – how they can and do work together – makes a big difference to what they're capable of. And this is often how it is with what your brain is doing.

Here's why this is all relevant: when it comes to mental health problems, it's common for people to wonder which part of the brain is going wrong. You may have bought this book with that exact question in mind. And it's perfectly reasonable, because if you know which part or bit of the brain is going wrong, surely there's a greater chance that it can be fixed? However, despite how reasonable and common this assumption may be, it's often wrong. Because it's a hugely overly simplified idea of how the brain works.

To wonder which bit of the brain is going wrong in, for instance, depression suggests that there is a low-mood-regulating centre or region of the brain, a bit that's solely responsible for the creation and maintenance of mood, that's somehow gone wrong. And there isn't, not really. Your mood

107

is a very complex, diverse experience, with multiple parts of the brain working together, or even against each other, and it's the more dominant processes that determine how you feel. To focus on which one bit is going wrong ignores all this, and that doesn't help us deal with the problem in hand.

Of course, just to make it more baffling, sometimes it *is* possible to trace a problem to a single part of the brain. For instance, we know which bit of the brain is going wrong in Parkinson's disease. It's the *substantia nigra*, a small but very important bundle of brain cells found deep in the lower levels of the brain. Sometimes, for reasons we're not one hundred per cent sure about, it starts to degrade and die. And then you get Parkinson's disease.[6]

Granted, Parkinson's disease is a neurological disorder, not a mental disorder per se, although it does invariably result in many mental health problems, like depression and mood swings, impulse control issues, and so on. But even so, the fact that Parkinson's can be attributed to physical disruption to a specific part (or parts) of the brain is one of the things that differentiates it from mental disorders. A neurological disorder is where there is a known disruption to the brain or nervous system; a mental or psychiatric disorder doesn't necessarily have this. It's sort of like a hardware versus a software problem.

Although even here, the distinction isn't completely clear. Surely everything involving our mind involves our brain? And if our mind starts doing unhelpful or disruptive things, doesn't this mean a part of the brain is doing something it shouldn't? Arguably, yes. That's undoubtedly why Parkinson's disease and other neurological disorders invariably feature mental health issues too. But there's a difference between problems caused by damage to the brain and nervous system, and problems caused by the brain and nervous system responding or adapting to things in negative ways. We'll explore more of this in later chapters.

Even if we *do* know which part of the brain is going wrong and causing mental or neurological problems, it doesn't mean dealing with them is any simpler. As stated, every bit of the brain is linked to pretty much every other one, often in alarmingly baffling ways. And certain parts of the brain regularly have multiple, diverse functions. Thus, even if a problem *begins* in one region, the effects and disruption that result from it spread, almost immediately, to countless other parts and processes.

You know when you put a load of 'whites' into the washing machine for a boil wash, but accidentally put a bright red sock in there too? It's a staple of sitcoms and cartoons. When this happens, you can identify the problem: the red sock. You can even stop everything and remove it from the washing machine. But that doesn't mean you've *fixed* anything. The other garments are still pink, because all the intense sloshing around has already happened. And so it is with certain parts of the brain: even if you could identify and fix the original problem, you still have to deal with the fallout, the bigger picture.

This impenetrable interconnectedness of the human brain and all the parts that make it up is a big part of what makes it so powerful and adaptable, but it also means there are countless ways for something to go wrong, and makes it damned hard to fix. This same applies to Huntington's disease, which I discussed earlier; it may be just one gene, just one protein, but that one protein interacts with hundreds of others in intricate, delicate chemical ways. Something going wrong with a certain part of the brain is the same thing, but on a larger, organic scale, not on the smaller, molecular one.

But whatever level you're at, the immediate issue is the same: how are you supposed to trace a problem, or do anything about it, when every part of the brain is connected to nearly every other part, of which there are thousands? How do you explore or adjust a part of the brain without risk of causing serious disruption or damage to all the other parts it's connected to? The simplest answer is, usually, you can't. Not with any thoroughness, anyway. The complex connections that make up the brain mean that anything can affect anything else. A drug may fix the main problem it's meant to deal with, but the presence of the drug could throw many other working systems out of whack. Hence, we have side effects.

However, those in the mental health field have to work with the limited tools they have to hand. A lot of the time, it comes down to a decision as to whether the effects of the mental health problem are more debilitating than the effects of the available treatment. Surprisingly often, the answer is no. A lot of drugs and other interventions don't make it through testing for these reasons, and patients often get their medications switched when one proves to be particularly unbearable.

That's another thing – as stated earlier, the human brain varies so much from person to person, because it forms and adapts to the things it experiences, and we all experience different things as we develop. But one result of this is that we tend to respond to drugs and treatments in different ways. That's why you never get a guaranteed-to-work treatment of any particular mental health problem, something that is equally and reliably effective for everyone who experiences it. It's just not going to happen.

Essentially, everything that happens in the brain is like the famous butterfly of chaos, flapping its wings and causing hurricanes several continents away. Except it's hundreds of thousands of butterflies and hurricanes happening every second, but localised entirely within your skull. And trying to identify the root cause of a mental health problem can be like trying to find the butterfly by studying the movements of a specific hurricane, and working backwards from there. This is an almost impossible task in any case, and even if you find the butterfly and swat it, the hurricane isn't necessarily going to go away.

Brain software vs brain hardware

So, there we have what is essentially a whistle-stop tour of the workings of the brain. Tiny sparks in the membranes of neurons allow them to send signals and communicate with each other, via the release of neurotransmitters, which add a great deal of complexity to the proceedings. These processes depend on the smooth running of the molecular systems that keep a neuron alive and allow it to function, and genetic problems can introduce issues even at this deep level.

Neurons come in all shapes and sizes and abilities, and certain types combine and link up to create certain brain regions that do certain things. But the versatile and flexible nature of the brain's make-up means it can change and adapt, and everything can be interconnected, combining multiple different parts to form networks that are capable of baffling functions and actions. This complexity and flexibility, combined with our – even now – limited science, means we're still a long way off from understanding exactly how and why the interactions of microscopic brain cells give rise to something as complex and intricate as the human mind, or consciousness.

But it happens, whether we understand it or not. Unfortunately, this means that, a lot of the time, problems with the mind can't necessarily be traced to the physical systems in the brain going awry.

And here's another important point to end on. I mentioned it earlier, but it warrants repeating because it's so often overlooked. Sometimes it's very difficult, even impossible, to isolate which bit of the brain is going wrong in a mental health problem – but it could be the case that there's *nothing going wrong with the brain at all.* The brain can be working just fine, objectively speaking, but it's working fine at doing things that aren't helpful, or that are actively harmful.

So, yes, I will be focusing on the brain in this book, and the mental health problems I'll be covering can be, and often are, understood in terms of what's happening in the brain of the person experiencing them. I find this can help to ground understanding of mental health issues in a more tangible, universal way, which is the whole point of this book. But this doesn't mean there's automatically something wrong with the brain of the individual experiencing the issues. Their brain is usually fine, it's just doing stuff that, ideally, it would not do.

This might sound a bit confusing, but remember when I said it was like a hardware versus a software problem? And how you don't disassemble the computer if it gets a virus? Because it's working fine, it's just been given instructions it shouldn't have, and ended up doing disruptive things. This is what I was getting at with that analogy.

Basically, while it can be the case that a mental health problem is down to something going wrong in the brain, it could just as likely be due to the brain developing or adapting in ways that mean it ends up doing things that are unpleasant, unhelpful and disruptive, such as producing too much anxiety, or not changing negative moods, when the situation calls for a different approach. Admittedly, from the perspective of the person experiencing the mental health problem, the distinction isn't really a useful one. The end result is the same for them. But it is a useful distinction when it comes to understanding and, ideally, dealing with the problems.

If the brain's not working as it should, if it's been damaged or disrupted, how do we fix that? Can we get in there, with drugs or other medical approaches, to undo the damage? If the brain is working, but doing unhelpful things, how do we change what it's doing? Can we give it new instructions, via CBT or similar, to stop it doing those unhelpful things?

Our options may be limited, but it doesn't mean we have none. And the brain being the brain, it's often the case that it's both not working *and* doing the wrong thing, simultaneously. And it's so flexible that maybe psychotherapy can fix an underlying physical issue, like people with Parkinson's being coached to handle their movement better. And maybe drugs can help, even when there's no underlying physical cause. Many drugs are prescribed largely to deal with harmful symptoms in any case, while doing nothing about the root cause, where it's known. This also shows why sticking rigidly to one model of mental health is likely to be too narrow a focus, limiting options for helping overall.

So, the brain is extremely flexible, versatile, and ludicrously complicated. This can, and does, make it very hard to establish what exactly is going wrong when mental health problems occur. Sometimes, it's the brain's responses to things that cause the issues in the first place. But, on the other hand, the innate properties of the brain also give us a wider range of options and possible interventions than we could otherwise expect, and allow us to tackle issues in multiple ways, given how the brain responds to pretty much everything.

Is this a worthwhile trade-off, though?

Well, let's find out . . .

3: Depression

If you mention mental health or mental illness to most people, the first thing they'll think of is depression. Indeed, much of the discussion and debate around mental health stems from depression, or centres around it. Even the controversies around mental health tend to be depression-centric, like whether antidepressants are effective, or accusations of laziness and other grim stigmas, or the worrying number of people who insist it's something you can snap out of. Much of this stems from people's perception of depression.

In fairness, there are good reasons for depression hogging so much of the much-needed – but still insufficient – attention and awareness that mental health receives. Extensive statistical analysis shows that depression is the most common mental health problem worldwide,[1] followed by anxiety, schizophrenia and bipolar disorder. Some data show that between three per cent and ten per cent of the population are affected by depression. That, in fairness, is quite a wide range. There are reasons why it tends to be so unspecific, and we'll get to those later, but even if it's at the very lower end of the possible range, three per cent of literally everyone? That's still a staggering number of people. In the UK, it would mean that two million people, at the very least, live with depression in some shape or form.

That's enough for a decent-sized city. A city of depression.*

Data also show that depression is the second biggest cause of years lived with disability worldwide.[2] What does that mean, exactly? Well, it's a useful unit for measuring the overall burden, for a society, of a disease or health problem. You basically measure how common it is in any given population, as in what percentage of people tend to have this problem, and multiply that by how much it affects health, as in how incapacitating it is. The result is the years lived with disability score.

Because depression is both very common and frequently very debilitating, it scores very highly here. The only thing that scores higher is lower back pain, a condition that's both seriously debilitating, as it can make it practically impossible to even move, and also very common, given how it can be caused by something as innocuous and everyday as sitting still for too long, or a particularly powerful sneeze. Trust me on this.

Also, if invoking the stats and data doesn't resonate with you, here's a more personal perspective. My own life has been directly shaped by depression, multiple times, which I think shows both how common and how significant depression is.

My first foray into the media was writing about depression. Google 'Dean Burnett, Blue Monday'. It's hilarious. My personal investment in the issue was, undeniably, powerfully influenced by witnessing the reporting on a series of related

---

* I'm 100% certain that anyone from the UK reading the words 'city of depression' immediately had a specific place in mind. Possibly several.

incidents in my home town. Google 'Bridgend suicide incidents'. It is absolutely not hilarious in any way, shape or form. My breakout article that got me noticed was about depression, in the context of the tragic passing of Robin Williams, and that's why I write books like this now.

My life has been affected by depression, in one form or another, multiple times, even though I've *never actually experienced it myself*. It would also be fair to say that much of my career has been dedicated to pointing out how depression doesn't work like how it's often portrayed. So, how *does* depression work? What's going on in your head that results in this very common, but still very serious, mental condition?

Depression: what it *is,* what it *isn't*

Let's get one thing clear right now: depression is not just a bad or negative mood. It's partly that, in a way, but also considerably more. A bad mood, in this instance, is the mother and father of all understatements.

I've said this multiple times, in many different contexts, but I'm going to keep on saying it until it's no longer true: we really should have different words for standard, everyday depression and full-on clinical depression. At present, you can legitimately say you're depressed when you're in a bad or low mood, or if you're sad about something unpleasant happening to you, like losing your job, or a relationship breaking down. And that's fine. It's good and right to be sad, depressed, in situations like this.

117

But it's not the same as being depressed in the psychiatric or clinical sense, where you're in a literally debilitating mental state, lacking any discernible motivation or energy, and seemingly can't do anything about it. Being depressed when life deals you a devastating blow means your brain is responding appropriately to something that's happened. You're expressing the correct emotional reaction needed to process and, hopefully, deal with it. In many ways it's a healthy thing. It should be happening. It may not be pleasant or enjoyable, but that's just how it goes with health sometimes. A broken bone slowly knitting itself back together is seldom a fun experience, but it's a very good thing, nonetheless.

In contrast, being deeply depressed for no discernible reason, for very long periods, is an unhealthy thing, by most professional measures. If you go by the ICD or DSM, a depressive episode, as it's known, has several signature features. The low-mood state should be there, obviously, but it should be abnormal for the individual. Because we all have highs and lows in our life, and some people seem to just gravitate to low moods by default, for whatever reason. We all know somebody who seems permanently grumpy; the eternal pessimists who find the downside in every situation. That's just how some people are. It's normal for them. But a mood disorder is something that goes significantly beyond that, to the point where it's really out of character.

This atypical depressed mood must also last for two weeks at the very least, and should be present for most of the day, for almost every day, in this period. There should be no obvious cause for this mood, such as an existing physical illness or the presence of drugs or narcotics.*

Another key feature of depression is becoming uninterested in doing or experiencing things that usually bring you pleasure; or the inability to enjoy such things, even if you can bring yourself to engage in them. This deficit in pleasure is often termed anhedonia. There's also a marked and significant loss of general energy levels, and/or an increase in fatiguability, meaning you become very tired, very quickly and easily. You might argue that these are the same thing expressed in different ways, and many would agree with you, but as we've seen, each person and their symptoms can be relatively unique, so it's important to cover all bases.

These features – two weeks minimum of severely low mood with no obvious physical cause, loss of interest and experience of pleasure, and loss of energy levels – are the key elements needed for a diagnosis of depression.

There are plenty of other common symptoms, though, and at least four of the following must be present to confirm a depression diagnosis:

- Severe loss of confidence or self-esteem, and feelings of inferiority.
- Excessive and objectively unreasonable feelings of self-reproach and guilt.

---

* This isn't to say that you can't experience depression in such circumstances, because of course you can; it's just labelled and dealt with differently.

- Suicidal ideation, meaning persistently thinking about death and suicide.
- Impaired ability to think, concentrate or make decisions.
- Psychomotor impairment, meaning you become less co-ordinated and active.
- Any type of sleep disturbance.
- Changes in appetite and corresponding weight change, with it going either up or down.

There are other symptoms that can occur, but these are the main ones, at least as far as the psychiatric approach is concerned. Granted, even though the range of symptoms taken into account seems quite comprehensive, there are still many who argue, with good reason, that this clinical diagnostic approach is too limiting, and depression can take many other diverse forms. However, we covered that issue in the previous chapter, so for now let's focus on the fact that this clearly shows just how radically different the genuine mood disorder of depression is to the everyday experience of being sad or unhappy. And yet, both can be – and often are – described using the term depressed.

Using the same term for both occurrences can be a problem, not just because it can make discussions a bit tricky, but because you often get people conflating the two, thinking they're the same. We've already discussed how language can directly influence how people think about and perceive something, so this means that if someone's been depressed in the everyday sense, they often seem to think they know what it's like to be medically depressed. This can lead to the sorts of behaviours and comments from others that – even if they're completely well meant, with the best of intentions – can be a constant source of stress, anger and stigma for those who deal with serious depression on a regular basis. Things like telling people they should 'cheer up' or 'snap out of it', or 'try going for a walk, or get some exercise', or 'think positive', or 'count your blessings', or 'other people have it worse, you know' and so on and so on.

Let's be generous and assume the people who say these things genuinely believe they're helping. And, in fairness, if you're in a low mood or in a funk after going through some hard times, all these suggestions may well be useful when it comes to bringing you out of it. But they won't be much use when you have a genuine clinical condition. If anything, they can make it worse, because as well as the issues caused by the depression itself, you're constantly having to deal with these interjections from people who often get angry or upset with you when you don't follow their advice, or you try to explain to them why it's not helpful.

To show what I'm on about, here's Martha Mills, a social media manager who has experienced a lot of this stigma and unsolicited advice . . .

I still feel very awkward and embarrassed going to collect my prescription from Boots, which is silly, it's really, really silly, but I still do. I resent it, I feel myself tensing up when I know that my prescription is running out. It's on auto-repeat, so I just have to go and get it from them, but I hate having to do it. I feel awkward when I'm there, I feel

121

embarrassed and shove it in my bag as quickly as possible. It's a box of pills that's already in a little paper bag – lots of people are in there getting various prescriptions and bits and bobs, but for me, it feels the same as going and buying thrush cream or something like that. It's like 'Oh, I know what I need to do, I just really don't want to be doing this.' It's quite indicative of the stigma it gets, that I still don't feel very comfortable necessarily with the fact I have depression and that it is a major thing in my life and I have to rely on these tablets. I'd just like that to not be a thing.

The other things that are generally annoying are the people with their really helpful suggestions. It's incredibly tiring, trying to be polite to them about it, because they mean so well. But many of them don't have a clue. Some of them have maybe experienced a depressive episode following a period of grief or a job loss, and while that's entirely valid, it's not the same as somebody like myself, where doctors have gone 'I don't know why you got it, you just have. It could be genetic. We don't know.'

If it baffled them, then Joe Bloggs on the street or someone on Twitter telling me 'Oh, well I did this and it really helped, I changed my diet and it really helped,' isn't going to be much use. I'm glad it worked for them, but whatever I eat, whatever I do, I still want to throw myself in front of a bus, unless I'm medicated.

As Martha states, the problem is that these people do not know what it's like to be clinically depressed, any more than they'd know what someone who's lost a limb is experiencing because they once had a paper cut.

Luckily, thanks to all the awareness-raising efforts, clinical depression is becoming a better-acknowledged concept. More people than ever recognise that depression is a genuine health problem, not just a typical bout of sadness that everyone gets, and people aren't just too lazy or self-indulgent to work through it. Such accusations are still bleakly common, but they seem less common than they used to be, which is something.

But then, this mainstream normalisation (for want of a better word) of depression can be a mixed blessing. Anything complicated that is portrayed in the mainstream usually ends up being rather oversimplified and inaccurate, and that's often the case here. There are a lot of modern portrayals of depression that weirdly romanticise it, depicting it as an intense but fleeting burst of passionate sadness, or beautiful people being moody and distant in a somewhat cool way, or something that causes great torment but furious creativity in artistic types.

Human Resources Officer Lowri Williams has some interesting views on the clash between mainstream media and reality when it comes to portrayals of mental health . . .

The romanticised version of a girl having a depressive episode is probably where she's wearing a large oversized sweater, probably with nothing underneath it but some white slouch socks. It will be off the shoulder and she'll be holding a steaming mug of something and should be sat in a window seat, reading something, hair tousled or in a loose ponytail. That's the image of depression that is allowed. You're allowed to sit there and be introspective and quiet and reading and looking out of the window, it's that image you portray. It's beautiful, and sexy.

But in reality, if you're a large girl wearing an oversized sweatshirt, it's because that's the only sized sweatshirt that fits you, and it's the only thing you can find on your floor of crap in your bedroom, that doesn't have cat hair on it and you're only wearing nothing on the bottom because your leggings got holes in them or you just can't be bothered to find them.

You're not reading a book, you're reading the back of a – and I found myself doing this the other day – I read the cooking instructions on the back of a food packet five times. The food was in the oven burning because I just found myself reading and I was like, this is what introspective reading is. I'm never going to put an Instagram post of me doing that. I had a steaming mug of hot chocolate that I poured a large measure of bourbon in, and I was like, this is the reality.

Also, I've lost count of the number of complaints I've heard about the clichéd use of the head-clutcher image in articles about mental health. You know the one, the melancholy photo of someone with their head buried in their hands that sits atop countless mental health think pieces, particularly those that focus on depression. In fairness, as someone who has written many articles about depression for mainstream platforms, there are very few useful options available when it comes to showing pictures of mental health. We just had a whole chapter explaining how one of the main problems with mental health is that you can't see it, so taking a photograph of it is obviously a challenge. But still, it's something of a cliché now, automatically equating mental health issues, and depression in particular, with constant, debilitating misery.

And that's not a great approach, because, as I just mentioned, depression is so much more complicated than merely a prolonged period of sadness.

So, what do we know about depression? At least insofar as the latest science, at the time of writing, is concerned.

Disorders of the mood

To begin with, depression is categorised as a mood disorder. As the name suggests, the main feature of these is disruption or debilitating disturbance of an individual's mood. Just so we're all on the same page, mood here means your overall emotional state. Your mood is more long-term, but less specific, than individual emotional experiences. Moods are normally described in broader terms of positive or negative valence. In plain English, this means moods can be good, or bad, or sometimes neither. But you can still experience a range of emotions within a certain mood. You can be angry, frustrated, sad, exasperated, all palpably different emotions, but all of these can occur as part of a bad mood.

Also, moods and emotions can feed into each other in very complicated ways. For instance, if you're in a bad mood, you tend to be less sensitive or receptive to pleasant, enjoyable emotions, like those associated with laughter and contentment. We've all experienced those times when our favourite funny TV show or most beloved music, things that usually make us very happy, just seem annoying or frustrating, because we're 'not in the mood'. This suggests our moods dominate and influence our emotions.

But then, on the flip side, sometimes an unpleasant emotional experience can quickly put you in a bad mood, and a very positive one can bring you out of it. You can have a nightmare commute into work that puts you in a severely bad mood all morning, until your boss tells you you've just been unexpectedly promoted, at which point you're jumping with joy, all thoughts of road rage and traffic jams completely dismissed.

The point is, our emotions and moods have a huge impact on how we function. They are intertwined in very complex ways, and they can and do change readily, and often, in response to what's going on in our life at the time. Except, that is, for when you have a mood *disorder*. This, in essence, is where your mood changes in unhelpful, unpredictable, and often illogical ways, that have little or nothing to do with what's going on at the time. And, often most importantly, your mood won't change back. Your mood becomes detached from what's actually happening to you. And given the immense influence your mood has on how you think, act and perceive things, this can be a considerable problem.

It's also important to stress that mood disorders aren't limited to low mood. You can have the opposite too. High mood would be the logical term here, I guess. But we don't say that. We say *elevated* mood. Maybe because it sounds more technical? Or maybe because a brain being 'high' is already the term used to describe the effect of recreational drug use. Anyway, the point is, mood disorders can manifest via elevated mood, depressed mood, or cyclical mood, where mood changes between the two extremes.

Clinically serious cases of elevated mood are commonly described as mania, or hypomania, and it's where someone is persistently and seriously energised, erratic, giddy even. Their mood is most certainly elevated. While I won't be devoting a whole chapter to mania, I will dwell on it for a moment here, to emphasise a few important points. One is that, despite depression getting the lion's share of the attention, it is not the only mood disorder. It's just the most dominant one, because it's by far the most common.

Another thing to highlight is that there are those who describe mania as the mirror of depression, its polar opposite. While there are logical reasons for this, it's a potentially harmful claim if it leads people to think that, because depression brings you down and makes you unhappy, mania must bring you up and make you happy. True, there are often potent euphoric elements to episodes of mania, but it's regularly a serious issue with numerous severe consequences, so not really something to be embraced or celebrated. It's sort of like drugs of abuse; they do indeed provide a lot of pleasure for the user, but as everyone knows, that's far from *all* they do.

But still, stand-alone mania, where an individual experiences mania and nothing else, is comparatively very rare.

Indeed, data suggest that the vast majority of mania cases are found in bipolar disorder,[3] that combination of depression and mania, where an individual regularly swings from one extreme to the other. The fourth most common type of mental health problem, according to a lot of the data.

This is part of why the numbers around depression are so hard to narrow down. If you've got someone showing all the signs of depression, are they experiencing standard depression, or bipolar disorder? You could fill all the criteria for the former, then a few months later your behaviour changes radically and now it's clearly the latter. Yes, it makes things even more complicated yet again, where your diagnosis, something you may have spent years obtaining, can suddenly change. Another example of the limitations of the diagnosis model, I suppose.

The surprising variation of depression

Another complicating factor is that clinical depression can take a surprisingly wide variety of forms. It's not just a period of low mood.

Earlier on I listed the symptoms needed to be diagnosed with depression. Things like constant and unchanging low mood, loss of energy, insensitivity to pleasure-inducing things, suicidal thoughts, excessive guilt, and so on. However, I wasn't being completely thorough there. It's true that those symptoms are required for a diagnosis, but the diagnosis you'd get is for *major depressive disorder*. Specifically, if you have one confirmed episode, your diagnosis is major depressive disorder, *single episode*. If you have another one later, after recovering from the initial one, you have major depressive disorder, *recurring*.

Major depressive disorder is the most familiar and common type of depression. It includes all the classic features of depression portrayed in the mainstream: the bleak unchanging moods, the zero motivation, the unshakeable negative mindset, and so on. I also said earlier that there should be different words used for everyday depression and clinical, mentally unwell depression. To their credit, in the medical and psychotherapeutic worlds there clearly *are* different words for the different manifestations of depression and low mood. It's just unfortunate that such distinctions have yet to catch on in the wider world. But who knows, maybe given enough time, they will.

So, medically speaking, if you're going through a bad period because of some life event, you're said to be in a low mood. But if you're clinically depressed, you've got major depressive disorder, or one of the other clinically recognised types. We covered earlier why medical terms need to be as specific as possible, because you need to know what you're dealing with and how to go about it. Obviously, instances of depression and mood disorder are no exception.

But the wide range of possible symptoms indicates that there's a lot of variety to be found in depression, which means there are many different types and subtypes of depressive disorder. So much so, we won't be able to cover them all here, but here are a few examples.

There's psychotic major depression, where as well as all

the other familiar symptoms, the individual experiences psychosis, where they become delusional, sometimes even hallucinating. It seems like whatever issue is causing the depression is so potent that it's affecting the brain's ability to differentiate between what's real and what isn't, not just the ability to control and regulate mood.

There's melancholic depression, which is a lot like major depressive disorder, but even worse. The absence of or inability to experience pleasure is a core feature, but the individual is even less able to function overall. They tend to experience more severe weight loss, wake up a lot earlier, and their symptoms are typically much worse in the early hours too. This ties in to a lot of evidence that shows that depression and sleep are very intertwined.[4] Insomnia is a common feature in many types of depression. Our sleep is based on circadian rhythms, the patterns and intricate mechanisms by which our brains control when we're awake, tired, asleep, and so on. That's why you feel different levels of fatigue at different times of day. Sleep is a vital process for overall brain health, but these mechanisms for regulating it are easily thrown off at the best of times, by excessive stimulation or hormone imbalance, even light levels – hence we get jet lag.

But as the systems that regulate sleep are quite easily disrupted, and as whatever's causing depression is something that's throwing off the typical internal processes of the brain, in some cases depression causes a lack of sleep. A lack of sleep is even more taxing for the brain. Sleep is, among other things, where the brain consolidates existing connections, clears away waste and debris, and generally maintains all that's going on inside it. A sleep-deprived brain is less well maintained, meaning it has even less ability to counteract or stave off a mood disorder like depression. So, if depression causes sleep loss, a vicious cycle ensues. It would also mean symptoms vary based on time of day, as the chemical and neurological cycles that regulate sleep are peaking and troughing. This would help explain why melancholic depression is particularly severe and worse in the morning hours.

On the other side, there's dysthymia, which is where the symptoms of major depression are usually present, but are not quite as severe or debilitating, so the individual has a better chance of coping with it. The downside is, this milder variant tends to last a lot longer than the more severe depressive episodes, often enduring for two years or more. It's as if the individual here experiences a type of depression that isn't severe enough to be incapacitating, so their brains can keep working at something close to normal. But this results in a holding pattern, which isn't ideal. A serious depressive disorder can knock you flat, but this can force you to rest and get through it, to give your brain time to sort itself out, or maybe for you to seek help and intervention. Dysthymia doesn't push you to those extremes, but can linger for much longer as a result.

Unfortunately, sometimes the different types can team up, and you get double depression, which is long periods of milder dysthymia, punctuated by regular bouts of major depressive episodes. So, you have years where you're either quite depressed or seriously depressed.

Then we have the more specific types, like postpartum depression, which hits between ten and fifteen per cent of new mothers who have just given birth[5] (although some argue that it's considerably higher than this but that it isn't flagged up as a problem as much, because it's so common). It makes sense, unfortunately; after even the most textbook, problem-free birth, a woman has experienced substantial physical, hormonal and emotional upheaval, and now also has a tiny vulnerable human to care for, forever. It would be alarming if that *didn't* play havoc with their mental state.

There's also seasonal affective disorder, where people seem to experience regular bouts of depression, but only in the winter months. This could feed back into sleep and light levels. It's darker in the winter, there's less daylight, so the changes this causes to our delicate sleep systems could lead to depressive episodes. Or maybe it's just because winter means everything is bleaker outside, and if your mental health is already vulnerable, that could be enough to tip you over the edge.

You also get depression that is linked with some other health issue, like substance abuse, physical brain injury, or related neurological disorders like Parkinson's. It's quite common, for example, for people with a dementia diagnosis to also develop or show signs of depression. Dementia involves serious disruption to a wide range of the brain's workings, so the chances of the systems regulating mood being affected too are reasonably high. But even if they weren't, finding out you've got dementia is surely a traumatic experience – maybe even enough to push someone into a depressive state by itself. Indeed, diagnostic tests have been designed to help practitioners tell the difference between the dementia and depression.

That might sound a bit odd, because aren't they very different things? At the fundamental level, yes. But remember, mental or cognitive problems aren't things you can see directly; they're detected largely via observations of, and interactions with, a patient, usually via a range of tests and assessments. So, say you're giving someone a memory test to look for signs of dementia, and they get a very poor score; you could reasonably conclude that there's something wrong with their memory.

But what if they got a poor score because they have zero motivation for doing well on the test – because they genuinely think they're worthless and nothing matters? The poor test results would look the same, but the *cause* would be very different. And dementia and depression are treated very differently, so it's important to know what the actual problem is before you start suggesting medications and therapies.

Again, this isn't an issue unique to mental health problems; it's just more blatant there. For a more physical comparison, imagine if you went to the doctor because of your swollen ankles. Swollen ankles can be caused by sprain, obesity, or just old age, so the doctor gives them a cursory look and prescribes some painkillers, light exercise, or similar mild interventions. The problem is, swollen ankles are also a symptom of heart failure! Or kidney failure! Poor circulation from a weak heart can cause blood to pool and gather in the lower regions, causing swelling. The disrupted hormone and electrolyte balance caused by failing kidneys can also cause water retention and swollen ankles. It often looks the same from the outside.

If you present with swollen ankles, it's crucially important that your physician knows whether they're dealing with a minor physical injury or a collapsing vital organ. Similarly, if you present with poor scores on a memory test, it's vital that your doctor or therapist knows whether it's because of dementia or depression. Because dementia means a degeneration, a physical loss, of a wide range of brain areas. Depression means . . . something else.

And so, we get to the meat of the matter. What exactly is going on in the brain during an episode of depression? Why is it so disruptive, and how come it can affect us in such a wide range of ways?

The classic chemical imbalance theory

For many years, the dominant theory as to why and how depression happens was something called the monoamine hypothesis. This is fundamentally linked to antidepressants and how they work, so just a heads-up that we'll be discussing them in detail in this section.

This was mentioned earlier, but have you ever heard someone say that mental health problems are due to a 'chemical imbalance' in the brain? It's said often, although rarely explained in any detail. Where did this idea come from? In most cases, the answer to that is the monoamine hypothesis. Chemical imbalance is a simplistic way of describing it in layperson terms. But here's what it actually means.

Remember the last chapter, where we saw how import-ant neurotransmitters are to the brain? Your brain is totally dependent on these chemical messengers to do all that it needs to do. We also touched on the fact that there are many different types of neurotransmitters. They're usually defined by what class of chemical they belong to, rather than what they do, per se, because many neurotransmitters have a wide range of roles in the brain.

So, one class of neurotransmitters are the monoamine class. They're chemicals with a single amine molecule in-cluded in their structure.* Monoamine neurotransmitters are also the ones you're most likely to have heard of in the every-day world. Dopamine is a monoamine. As are noradrenaline and adrenaline, which are sort of the neurotransmitter and hormone versions, respectively, of the same thing.†

Dopamine is often labelled a 'happy chemical', due to its crucial role in the experience of reward and pleasure, which is something we'll get to later. The same is true of serotonin, which might sound familiar because of its central role in the treatment of depression. You may have heard, for instance, of SSRIs: selective serotonin reuptake inhibitors. Prozac, Zoloft, Luvox; these common antidepressants are all SSRIs.

Actually, let's step back a bit.

* If you want to know precisely what this means, please consult the nearest professional chemist, because this is beyond my remit. But for now, let's just accept that monoamines are a certain type of neurotransmitter.

† Readers in the States and other countries may know adrenaline and noradrenaline as epinephrine and norepinephrine. Same thing, different labels. Because neuroscience isn't confusing enough already.

Antidepressants as we know them were discovered in the late 1940s and 1950s, largely by accident.[6] The first antidepressants began life as experimental drugs for other ailments, like tuberculosis and surgical shock, a condition caused by disruption to blood flow after operations. But researchers soon realised these experimental substances caused patients' moods to elevate, making them happier and more energised, and wondered what was going on. And lo, antidepressants were born.

I could go on about the specific mechanisms and chemical nature of these antidepressants, invoking terms like tricyclic amines and monoamine oxidase inhibitors, but that would get confusing very quickly. However, the main effect of all these antidepressants was that they increased the activity of monoamine neurotransmitters in the brain, most commonly by preventing the neurotransmitter from being removed from the synapse.

We've seen how a neurotransmitter works, how it allows the passage of signals from one neuron to another across the synapse. But when a neurotransmitter is released into a synapse, it doesn't just linger there indefinitely. It's a chemical messenger; leaving it there means it would keep repeatedly 'delivering' the message. And if that message is 'activate, create signals!' then the recipient neuron will keep activating and sending signals, long after it needs to.

It's like someone not taking their foot off the accelerator in a car when it's hit the desired speed. That's unhelpful, for many reasons. So, once they've done what they need to do, neurotransmitters are usually broken down into ineffective components, removed by other mechanisms, or reabsorbed back into the neuron to be used again later. It varies depending on which neurons or transmitters you're talking about, but in any case, they're got rid of.

Essentially, the original antidepressants prevented this neurotransmitter removal from happening. Or at least slowed it down somewhat. They caused neurotransmitters to linger longer in the synapses, continuing to have their effects, increasing the overall stimulation of the recipient neurons. But only for certain monoamine neurotransmitters, like noradrenaline, or more typically these days, serotonin.

So, antidepressants were, and still mostly are, chemicals that increase the activity of monoamine neurotransmitters in the brain. This often causes depressed patients to feel better, and to regain normal functioning. Therefore, it was concluded that depression comes about when your brain doesn't have enough monoamine neurotransmitters, for whatever reason. And so, the monoamine hypothesis of depression was born. As a result, the monoamine systems of the brain have been the main target for antidepressant drug research for decades. And given the logic that those with depression lack the normal, required levels of certain important chemicals, that's where the whole chemical imbalance explanation of depression, and many other mental health issues nowadays, stems from.

It's all nice and neat when you think about it, isn't it? Unfortunately, it's *too* neat.

The monoamine hypothesis has fallen out of favour in recent years,[7] because as the data build up, a lot of problems with it have arisen. The most obvious one is this: let's assume that depression genuinely is caused by harmfully low levels of monoamine neurotransmitters, like serotonin, and this is the root cause of depression. This is a not unreasonable interpretation of the monoamine hypothesis. So, if this is the sole cause of depression, then increasing the presence of serotonin to more normal levels should be all you need to do to resolve the depression, yes?

Here's the issue: given the speeds at which our bodies operate at the chemical level, the important substances in antidepressants enter our bloodstream and get to work in our brains in a matter of minutes. Antidepressants are increasing the presence of serotonin in your neurons pretty much as soon as you've taken them. So, logically, we should see antidepressants working pretty much immediately. Except, *we don't*. Even the most reliable antidepressants can take several weeks before having any therapeutic benefit. What gives?

The thing is, we know they're doing *something*, because the side effects usually kick in pretty quickly. Remember, neurotransmitters perform multiple functions throughout the brain and body. If you alter the levels of them with drugs, it'll affect multiple systems, and a lot of those effects won't be great. So, we can be sure that antidepressants are indeed boosting serotonin or other neurotransmitter levels from the get-go, but the depression itself isn't being affected. Weird, right?*

---

* These numerous side effects are also why tolerability is a big concern when manufacturing and prescribing drugs, particularly psychoactive ones.

And here's an interesting fact: the most common anti-depressants – the SSRIs like Prozac – are not actually the best at tackling depression.[8] Compared to other drugs, their effect on depression is relatively mild. Amitriptyline is the most reliably potent antidepressant, according to the data, and that's one of the oldest types of antidepressant, of the tricyclic amine class.

So, why are SSRIs far more common when more effective types are available? It's because more potent drugs also have more severe side effects, such as constipation, dizziness, migraines, even heart and kidney issues. SSRIs have side effects too, of course, but they are comparatively less common and/or less severe. Fewer people experience a bad reaction to SSRIs than any other antidepressant, according to the evidence. And that often makes them a best first choice.

Basically, a drug that tackled depression reliably every single time would be great, but what if it gave you constant stomach cramps, insomnia, rapid heart rate and liver failure? Many patients would consider that as debilitating as the depression, or even worse. So, what would be the point of it? Indeed, there are many drugs like this, which are usually reserved for treatment-resistant depression, a manifestation of depression where, as the name suggests, typical treatments don't seem to have much impact. In cases like this, where the depression is particularly bad and stubborn, the more potent drugs are brought out, because the individual may well be willing and able to live with the side effects if it means regaining control of their moods.

139

Again, though, it bears repeating that people react differently to each drug, and the side effects will be more or less debilitating depending on who you are and what your life involves. Girl on the Net, an anonymous sex blogger, has a good example of this.

> *After I got my diagnosis, my doctor prescribed me sertraline to basically help make me feel a bit better. I found out later that apparently the dose they gave me was quite high but at the time, the thing that frustrated me most about it is I specifically asked my doctor about side effects and they said, 'Oh no, there won't really be that many, you might feel a little bit fuzzy.'*
>
> *What they didn't mention was that it made me completely unorgasmic the whole time I was taking it. At no point was that mentioned to me and so I stopped taking it after a few months. Some people don't mind that as a side effect or it bothers them less, but I'm a sex blogger and writer. For me, that is the core rich seam of joy in the middle of my life, which was being completely shut down. I couldn't orgasm through sex or masturbation. It didn't make me depressed as such – I don't know what it made me because I was on SSRIs – but it made me very sad.*

But back to the original point: if increasing the presence of monoamine neurotransmitters doesn't help depression right away, there must be more to it than that. The thing is, since the discovery of antidepressants, our understanding of the brain and our ability to investigate its workings have increased drastically. And this, as with most scientific en-deavours, calls earlier conclusions into question. In this case, the conclusion – that the root cause of depression is having insufficient neurotransmitters like serotonin – is constantly being shown to be at best a drastic oversimplification, if not plain wrong.

For example, serotonin neurons and their connections have long been implicated in mood regulation, hence SSRIs are so common. And it was widely assumed that the serotonin system in the brain was one big network, starting in the brainstem, the most fundamental layer of the brain, then branching out extensively into many other areas of the brain, which would explain why serotonin-based medication is reliably effective. However, studies published as recently as 2018 revealed evi-dence that suggests there are at least two *separate* serotonin systems in the brain.[9] Furthermore, the data suggest there could be several more that haven't yet been identified.

What's the significance of this? One network, two, twelve, fifty, what does it matter? It matters in this case because the two separate serotonin systems identified seemingly have different, *opposing* effects on mood. Activation of one system seems to boost signs of good mood and motivation, while activation of the other system made subjects (in this case, mice) appear more anxious and nervous, or display other animal equivalents of depression.

There are many instances of people having negative or unhelpful reactions to SSRI antidepressants. It's a small per-centage of the number of people who actually take them, but it's still been flagged up by regulatory bodies that SSRIs can sometimes increase your depressed mood, or even make you experience more suicidal ideation. This can be especially true for younger patients, or those who are in the first few weeks of taking them.

Why would this happen? How could a drug widely prescribed because it elevates your mood have the opposite effect in certain people, despite being the exact same molecule? Well, there's the fact that every brain develops differently because we all have unique lives and unique internal environments. Also, the specific cellular workings of the brain are endlessly complex and nuanced. So, what if in most people it's the good mood serotonin system that is boosted by SSRIs, while in other people, or in earlier stages of the medication, it's the bad mood one that is more responsive to the elevated serotonin levels caused by the medications, leading to worse moods and side effects?

Maybe it's not the chemical balance that's being thrown off, but rather the balance between the levels of activity in the matching, but *opposing*, serotonin neural networks that influence mood, both of which use the same neurotransmitter? To put it in more relatable terms, think of it like running a bath. You have a hot and a cold tap, right? Matching, but opposing. And when used together properly, they do their job well. But then you check the bath and find it's not filling up fast enough, and you turn one tap so it's pumping out more water.* Except,

* A quick aside for American readers: unlike your own plumbing preferences, it's typical in the UK to have two faucets – one for hot water, and one for cold. I guess the analogy still works if it's one faucet with two dials, but I don't think it's as good then.

what if you don't know which tap is which? You could end up with a full bath that's freezing cold, and that's no good.

Maybe boosting serotonin levels in your brain when you don't know which system you're influencing is like that: randomly turning the taps in hope of a hot bath. There's no guarantee you won't make things worse.

Again, be aware that while this may *sound* reasonable, it is an extrapolation on my part, based on very new data. Over the coming years, research may well uncover new aspects and variables that explain things even more thoroughly. Basically, this information about different serotonin systems is so new that we've not had time to investigate it yet. I'm just highlighting how advances in information can change accepted wisdom and help explain previously mysterious things.

I also mention all this to demonstrate how easy it can be to create robust-sounding ideas of how the brain works based on what is, when you step back and look at it honestly, a rather limited amount of information. So, while simple and straightforward explanations like the monoamine hypothesis are very appealing, the way the brain works almost inevitably means the bigger picture will be something far more complex.

Here's another issue with the monoamine hypothesis. If the whole thing rests on the conclusion that depression is caused by unhelpful changes to the levels of monoamine in the brain, how do you explain the fact that there are some effective antidepressants out there that *don't* affect mono-amine transmitter levels at all? If the power company tells you that you've got no electricity because of problems with

143

the grid, but you replace a fuse and all the lights come back on, doesn't that mean the power company was wrong? It's a similar situation here. For a long time, experts believed that depression was caused by insufficient monoamines in the brain, but now we have antidepressants that tackle depression while leaving the monoamine levels untouched, because they work on other types of transmitters, like glutamate.[10]

Some could argue that maybe those alternative drugs are just masking the symptoms of depression, rather than fixing the problem? They're breaking out the candles and torches during the power cut, not actually addressing the underlying issue. But then, maybe *all* antidepressants do that? But given that it's a mood disorder, something almost entirely mental, and not a virus or something more tangible, maybe the symptoms are all you need to worry about?

And once again, we get bogged down in maybes and what-ifs. Such things are pretty much inevitable when you try to explain incredibly complicated neuropsychological processes in terms of simple chemical imbalances. The focus is far too narrow, too limited.

So, what else seems to be happening in the brain during depression?

Neuroplasticity: a new cause of depression?

With the increasing limitations of the monoamine hypothesis becoming ever more apparent, the search for an understanding of the neurological mechanisms of depression has branched out in several directions. One particularly interesting focus concerns neuroplasticity.[11] Neuroplasticity is essentially the brain's ability to change and adapt at the cellular level. It can reorganise itself, make new connections, remove ones it doesn't need, expand areas and processes that become more important over time, and shrink those it doesn't use so much any more. Such abilities are vital; the brain constantly needs to react, respond and adapt to all the things that happen to us. That's what it's for. Because the world around us is always changing, a static, fixed brain is no use. A static brain is inert. A static brain is dead.

For a long time, though, it was assumed the adult brain was essentially rigid, that once your development during childhood and adolescence was finished, that was it. Your brain stayed as it was for the rest of your life. However, recent findings show this to be wrong. True, the overall gross structure of your brain is largely set when you reach adulthood; the major pathways and networks are in place and it seems there's not a lot that can be done to rework or rearrange them. But there's still ample room for flexibility.

Think of it as if your brain is a house. As you grow and develop, the house that is your brain is still being built. Once you're an adult, it's done. You can't really do much about the walls or foundations at this point, but you can still redecorate, change the wiring, put in new windows, and so on. Maybe even add an extension or redo the plumbing? Such things can make big differences.

And such changes in the brain are possible, because neurons are plastic, as in *flexible*. They can change their shape, grow new connections or lose old ones, change their output

145

and signalling, their functioning, thanks to all those useful properties we covered earlier. Therefore, neuroplasticity is vitally important.

Except there's now a lot of evidence to show that, in people with depression, their brain's neuroplasticity is somehow diminished. The technical aspects are very complex, and nobody is one hundred per cent sure about exactly what's going on, but there are mounting data that strongly suggest a depressed brain is, in certain key areas, less able to change, and adapt, at the cellular level.

How would this result in depression? Well, remember that depression is described not so much in terms of someone being in a low or bad mood as when such moods become fixed. As in, someone falls into a very low mood, and can't come out of it; they can't change what their brain is doing. If you look at depression this way, as your underlying brain cells losing their usual ability to adapt, to change, it all suddenly makes a bit more sense.

At the start of this chapter, we saw how responsive and variable mood and emotion can be. But if your brain is less able to shift and adapt to new situations, your mood could essentially be locked. Of course, the brain doesn't completely lose the plasticity it needs to function; those with depression are still able to think and interact and move around, it's just that doing so is much harder than it should be. Which is probably what you'd expect if the brain cells responsible for all these things had lost some, but not all, of their give; as if they were mired in tar, or something.

Having said that, there are cases of catatonia in certain

146

extreme cases of depression, where individuals become even more irresponsive, barely moving or talking at all. Perhaps this is due to even greater loss of plasticity? To even more neurons becoming rigid and unresponsive?

In the last chapter I covered the many reasons why looking for a specific part of the brain responsible for disorders like depression was generally an overly simplistic and none too helpful approach. You'd expect a network of brain regions, many different parts operating together, to be involved in something as complex and variable as mood. If that's the case, in depression, wouldn't you expect to see impaired functioning, or reduced neuroplasticity, even shrinkage, in multiple brain areas? Yes. And this is pretty much what happens.

Several studies have revealed reduced size and activity in the hippocampus in depressed patients. The hippocampus is an integral and fundamental region of the brain for learning and memory, which means it's strongly linked to many other important areas. Some theorise that this reduction in hippocampal size and function explains why depression is so often associated with memory impairment,[12] something else that makes the dementia/depression overlap even more confusing. But it's also seen as causing a loss of *coping* ability, because you need to learn and retain new information to be able to cope and move on from unpleasant experiences and associated modes of thinking. An underperforming hippocampus would hinder this ability, and would also explain how those with depression cannot progress and move on from their low mood.

Other studies have found similar deficits in the prefrontal cortex, the high-level thinking brain regions behind the eyes,

147

responsible for our most complex and sophisticated cognitive abilities – abilities such as impulse control, the ability to evaluate and restrict your more fundamental, basic urges. Impairment of this ability is, according to many, the reason why those with depression can be vulnerable to suicidal ideation or other negative drives. If you're already prone to impulses to harm yourself, or worse, then the parts of your brain that think logically and rationally about risk and consequence are disrupted, this is a very bad combination. Also, decreased activity in these higher-reasoning areas would potentially explain why depression often makes it so difficult to just think clearly in general.

Other studies point to similar negative changes in the anterior cingulate cortex, a region located towards the centre of the brain, which essentially forms a collar around the corpus callosum, the white matter bridge that connects the two brain hemispheres. The anterior cingulate cortex is strongly implicated in processing and resolving negative emotions, among other things. Essentially, it allows us to feel the relevant feelings when something bad has happened, and make sense of them. Relatedly, this brain region also seems to be extensively linked to regulation of mood, to our ability to experience different moods in response to different situations and occurrences. Predictably, this region has received a lot of attention from those researching depression.

Other studies show reduced activity in another brain region, the striatum, and its subregions, including one named the ventral tegmental area. This is also located towards the centre of the brain, but more towards the core of the hemispheres, not at the edges like the anterior cingulate cortex. Reduced activity in the striatum is important because the striatum is heavily involved in human social behaviour, while the ventral tegmental area is a key element of the reward pathway, the part of the brain that allows us to feel pleasure. Maybe this explains the anhedonia, the inability to feel pleasure from things, experienced in depression. And maybe the lack of socialising drives, too?

Now, again, the caveat is that, while many of these findings have a lot of evidence to support their validity, in many cases you can find studies that say the opposite of what I've said here. It's always tricky to be sure what you're seeing when you're scanning a human brain, as there's just so much going on, and the results you get can be severely affected by the type of question being asked of your subject, and how you interpret the data. But let's assume for now these deficits of key brain regions are legitimate. One thing that would explain the lack of activity in these regions, and their reduced size, is if they had reduced neuroplasticity.

If the component neurons are less adaptable, less responsive, then you'd see less activity, less signalling from them, and a reduction in the number of connections and synapses they form, because all these things are sustained by constant activity. Therefore, you'd expect to see these affected brain regions getting quieter, and smaller, as they're taking up less space. So, neuroplasticity loss is a strong contender for the explanation of how depression happens.

But still, there are questions.

The drugs *do* work? Antidepressants and their mechanisms

If we accept that neurons losing their plasticity is the root cause of depression, and it's nothing to do with depleted levels of neurotransmitters, it then begs the question of why antidepressants, which raise neurotransmitter levels, would work at all. Because they do, much of the time. But here's the thing: it's wrong to say depression has *nothing* to do with neurotransmitter levels. If you have neurons that are less active and not as responsive, then they'd logically be releasing fewer neurotransmitters into synapses, which means lower neurotransmitter levels.

This also potentially explains why antidepressants take so long to kick in. In the context of depression being a result of lost neuroplasticity, it's argued that when antidepressants work, it's because they generate extra stimulation for inactive neurons, which 'wakes them up'. Neurons are essentially tiny microscopic factories, filled with molecular production lines churning out all manner of vital substances and signals, in order to do all they need to do. The theory is that in depression, the factory is slowing down, reducing production and output. It's been deprived of all but emergency power to keep things ticking over. Neuroplasticity has been lost.

But then along come antidepressants, and it could be that they basically start pumping the bellows, firing up the furnace, and so get the factory going again. But because it's so intricate and involves so many molecular steps, bringing up levels of plasticity is a gradual process; maybe it's less like flicking a switch, and more like fertilising and watering a parched plant. It may well recover and grow back, but it won't happen right away.

Of course, there are other explanations for the lengthy time antidepressants take to work. Some studies suggest that antidepressant chemicals have a variety of effects at the cellular level, some of which are helpful, some of which are disruptive, and it takes a while for all these to sort themselves out, and for the former effects to gain the upper hand. Others believe it's more to do with the cognitive process, in that the chemical effects are immediate, but our brain's ability to process positive emotional reactions takes longer to emerge from the overwhelmingly negative mindset a depressed person is currently dealing with. And so on.

Because it's the brain, it may be that all these explanations, and more, are part of what's really happening. It's a very diverse organ, to say the least. However, here's another thing to consider. The problem with antidepressants that work on the monoamine systems could be that, despite how well known and exhaustively researched they are, the monoamine systems are a surprisingly small part of the overall mass of our brains. This isn't to say they're unimportant, because they're clearly *very* important. But they're like the slender veins of minerals found in a hefty slab of marble, or the volume dial on a radio – crucial, but still a relatively small component of the overall system.

If you want to talk about the big daddy of stimulating neurotransmitters in the brain, you need to talk about the one mentioned in passing earlier. Glutamate. Most data show that glutamate makes up ninety per cent of the neuro-transmitter presence found in the brain's synapses at any one time.[13] It would take multiple books to cover everything that glutamate does in the brain, so I won't even try to do that here. Basically, while the brain uses many different neurotransmitters, in terms of actual raw numbers it's more of a 'glutamate . . . with special guests' scenario.

Here's why this is important. If we accept that antidepressants work by boosting neuroplasticity, then the commonly used monoamine antidepressants, like SSRIs etc. would only boost activity in very limited areas of the brain, in terms of the percentage of neurons they act on. However, depression affects many different, and widespread, areas of the brain.

This doesn't mean monoamine antidepressants won't work. They regularly do. Remember, every part of the brain is connected to every other, so if you boost activity in one select region – in this case certain monoamine systems, in-creasing neuroplasticity in the process – this raised activity will be gradually passed on to the connected regions further downstream.

Indeed, as mentioned already, many of the neurons that use serotonin, the most typical target of modern antidepressants, branch out from the brainstem, the most fundamental neuro-logical area, and spread throughout nearly all distinct regions of the brain. It's also worth noting that a typical effect of sero-tonin is to modulate neurons, to make them more sensitive to other transmitters. In essence, serotonin makes other neurotransmitters more effective, in widespread regions of the brain.

152

It's like a fantasy video game. Serotonin isn't the main character, tackling the quest, but the wizened old man with a stall, dispensing healing potions and power-ups just when needed. Not the hero, but making the hero's job easier. Hence, medications that enhance serotonin would be, and are, quite useful.

But still, even as widespread and helpful as they are, the serotonin or other monoamine neurons only represent a small part of what's going on in the brain. Let's say treating depression in the brain is like trying to restart a fire that's gone out. The kindling and fuel are all there, it's just no longer burning like it was previously. Using the more common antidepressants is maybe like trying to relight it by holding up a magnifying glass and focusing the sun's rays on a bit of kindling. It could work – odds are, it will. And it should spread to the rest of the fuel too. But it takes *time*. Focusing all efforts on one specific spot means the eventual success comes about via rather indirect routes.

Using monoamine-based antidepressants like SSRIs is like this. It's focusing on an important, useful, but still relatively small part of the brain's circuitry, and hoping the benefit spreads.

By contrast, look at ketamine. Often used as an anaesthetic or narcotic, because it packs a serious punch, ketamine is a tightly controlled and highly regulated substance, and for good reason. It's an incredibly powerful drug, with the potential to do severe damage if used carelessly. However, even when keeping all these dangers and risks in mind, there's currently a lot of buzz around ketamine's potential as

153

an antidepressant. What trials there have been have repeatedly shown it can be very effective in treating even serious, treatment-resistant depression.

And even more intriguingly, the effects can take just a few days, sometimes even just a few hours to kick in, rather than the weeks of more traditional antidepressants.[14] The reason for this is believed to be that ketamine works on glutamate receptors and neurons, those responsible for most of your brain's activity. Ketamine stimulates a lot more of your brain, so far more of the sluggish neurons get a proverbial kick up the backside to get them firing again, bringing neuroplasticity back to normal levels much faster. To go back to the example of relighting a fire, if SSRIs are using a magnifying glass to focus the sun's rays, ketamine is like dousing it all in petrol and throwing lit matches at it. Which would you expect to succeed first?

This may also explain why other psychedelic, hallucinogenic compounds, like LSD and those derived from magic mushrooms, are proving fertile ground for antidepressant research.[15] If they stimulate more of the brain, they're potentially having a quicker, stronger, and broader effect on reduced neuroplasticity.

Of course, this is a mixed blessing. If ninety per cent of your brain is being artificially stimulated, boosted, that's not automatically a *good* thing. We've seen that monoamine antidepressants, which focus on a much smaller number of neurons and systems, can still have unpleasant side effects. But ketamine is far more powerful, with more widespread actions across your brain. How bearable do you think *those* side effects would be?

But the obstacles of drug research aside, the case for impaired neuroplasticity being responsible for a lot of what happens in depression is increasingly compelling. More and more data are being generated that support the idea that reduced neuroplasticity is a root cause of much of what we see in depression, and other related disorders. Similarly, drugs that seemingly can and do counteract this plasticity loss, like ketamine and hallucinogens, are gaining ground as viable treatments for depression due to the therapeutic effects they have. Indeed, in March 2019, the FDA in America approved the use of the first ketamine-based antidepressant for patients with treatment-resistant depression. It's a nasal spray, interestingly enough.[16] Either way, it shows that the approach of using such drugs is becoming more common.

Heck, it doesn't even need to be drugs! Cognitive therapies can be quite effective, and we saw that they essentially work by helping the individual to think and process things in less disruptive or debilitating ways. Some argue that when therapists do this, they're raising neuroplasticity in the brain by causing patients to engage new, and hopefully less affected, neural systems, prompting increases in activity overall.

Another approach is brain stimulation, either with implanted electrodes or focused electromagnetic fields, and this is also showing promise as a viable treatment for depression.[17] Stimulate the brain in certain places, neuroplasticity elevates, the activity spreads, we know how this goes now. In theory.

Of course, if all else fails, there's the option of electroconvulsive therapy, ECT. Although this was given a severely bad reputation by the film *One Flew Over the Cuckoo's Nest*, which did for ECT what *Jaws* did for sharks, it is known to be a very effective treatment, albeit one that is not used unless absolutely necessary.[18] It makes sense, in this context; a powerful electrical current is passed through the brain, triggering a seizure. It's not exactly pleasant, and it's not without risks, but if anything is going to jump-start sluggish neurons . . .

In the restarting a fire example, ECT is strapping on a flame thrower and blasting everything with a white-hot blaze. Drastic, sure. Effective, certainly. But not without peripheral scorching and damage if you're not one hundred per cent careful. It's a bit like invasive surgery; even if it's completely successful and everything goes smoothly, the very act of opening someone up and rearranging their insides is still disruptive, so recovery and side effects are usually unavoidable.

So, you could say a clearer picture of depression is coming into focus. It may be something that occurs when the neurons in various parts of the brain lose their plasticity, their adaptability. Antidepressant therapies work by counteracting this – by coaxing, or forcing, the neurons back to normal activity, directly or indirectly.

Seems sensible. But, once again, there are still unanswered questions.

Stressing the important role of stress in depression

So, let's say depression is the result of parts of the brain losing plasticity, being underactive. Fair enough. But what of the data that say there are some brain regions that are *overactive* in depression? Because there seem to be quite a few. Most notably, these include the insular cortex, the orbitofrontal cortex and the amygdala.

The insular cortex is believed to be a key area for processing feelings of disgust, as well as having extensive connections to the deeper emotion-processing regions of the brain, so is implicated in feelings of self-worth and our overall emotional state. A brain region involved in both sense of self-worth *and* negative emotions, being overactive? Sounds like something that would result in depressive symptoms.

The orbitofrontal cortex is another higher-brain region involved in consciousness and thinking, and is most often referenced as an area that controls the more emotional, impulsive elements of the brain. Basically, the orbitofrontal cortex is usually the little angel on the shoulder that tells you not to do things, to resist baser urges. That's usually good, but . . . what if it goes too far? If the little voice in your head that says 'no' is too powerful, too persistent, it would drain your motivation to do anything. An overly active orbitofrontal cortex has been found to be present in things like sexual dysfunctions,[19] and you can see how such a thing would lead to the tremendous motivation drain seen in most cases of depression.

And finally, there's the amygdala, a well-known and heavily researched brain region. It's thought of as the hub of emotional processing, as it's seemingly the part of the brain that determines what emotional reaction is warranted in any given situation. It also adds the emotional content of memories, to reinforce what it's learned, thanks to its very close connections to the memory-processing hippocampus. However, most scientists focus on the amygdala's role in fear, and other negative emotions. Essentially, an overactive amygdala means more negative feelings and emotions. You might hope that your brain would learn that these feelings are unwarranted and stop them, but then what if the hippocampus, which supports learning, is compromised (as it is in depression, apparently)?

So, this raises questions. Why are some parts of the brain diminished in depression, presumably by a reduction of neuroplasticity, while some parts increase in their potency and output? How can there be an underlying cause of depression that has two opposing consequences, in different brain regions? Well, again, the nature of the brain means such a range of effects are well within its capabilities, but a lot of modern evidence points to one underlying factor.

Stress.

We all know the 'everyday frustrations of life' kind of stress, and that is a big part of this. But I also mean stress on a cognitive and cellular level. In essence, stress is the first stage of the fight-or-flight response, the deeply ingrained reflex that compels you to tackle dangers head-on or run screaming from them.*

But this potent fear response isn't like a switch, a simple yes or no thing. In fact, there are several neurological and biochemical systems that prepare your brain and body for

---

* There is also a third option included in the modern-day understanding of fight-or-flight: freeze, which explains that inability to move when you're truly scared.

having to deal with a threat. That process is, basically, what stress is. It's regulated by a complex suite of brain networks and hormonal reactions, and one key element in the stress response is the amygdala, the part of the brain that decides whether stress is warranted.

But it's the underlying mechanisms of it all that are intriguing here, because the stress response has numerous potent effects on us. It increases the focus and attention the brain pays towards negative things. Usually, this is whatever's causing the stress, because when you're dealing with a problem, you can't afford to waste time pondering irrelevant things, so your brain sticks to the important, and invariably negative, things you're experiencing.

Stress puts your brain and body into a more alert state, meaning you become more sensitive to hazards and risks, both physically and mentally. It's useful for keeping you safe but leads to you focusing on the negatives – the unpleasant aspects of your current existence – and downplays the potentially distracting positives.

Another big problem is that, because of these things, stress is very stimulating. This is true on a physical level as well; stress releases several potent chemicals into your bloodstream, such as cortisol, which amps up your heart rate, muscle tension, glucose uptake, even your immune system responses. That's why constant, prolonged stress can be physically harmful. And there's now a lot of evidence to show that stress is invariably a key factor in depression,[20] because the trigger, the activation of the stress response, comes from our brain – probably the amygdala, as we've seen. Wherever it originates, though, it has numerous knock-on effects, intended to bring everything else – all the required physical and neurological processes – in line, for a viable stress response. A key element is the hypothalamic-pituitary-adrenal (HPA) axis.[21]

This axis is essentially a complex association between the hypothalamus, and the pituitary and adrenal glands. Broadly speaking, all three are crucial areas found in different parts of the brain and body, but all are generally responsible for controlling the relationship between the nervous system and the endocrine system. In even simpler terms, they allow your brain to control what chemicals go into your body, and when, and why.

The HPA axis is basically the link between the brain and the body when it comes to stress. When our brain decides that stress is required, signals are sent to the HPA axis, which in turn releases a complex sequence of chemicals that ends up with stress hormones, like cortisol and glucocorticoids, being released into our bloodstream. This puts the body on alert, for want of a better description. It primes our physical systems for a fight-or-flight response, and usually lasts several hours, until the stress chemicals subside and our body returns to normal.

Now, here's the tricky part. The output of the HPA axis, this intricate chemical system that controls our physical responses to stress, is sort of self-regulating, via a complex feedback system. Basically, the axis that produces the stress chemicals also recognises when levels of these chemicals are too high, then shuts off the supply.

It's like a bathtub again. You turn the taps on when you need water, but when there's too much water and the whole thing is on the verge of overflowing, you turn the taps off. Both the taps-on and taps-off actions are determined by the level of water present, and similarly, both the stress-on and stress-off action of the HPA axis is determined by the levels of stress chemicals in the bloodstream. Hopefully, this makes sense.

But here's the problem: for some reason, in many a modern-day adult brain, this ability of the HPA axis to recognise when there's enough stress chemical in the body, and cease production, is disrupted in some way. Basically, the HPA axis can start the physical stress response, but doesn't seem to know when to stop. This might sound like a mild annoyance, but there's mounting evidence that suggests it's a cause of multiple mental health problems, particularly depression.[22] Those who suffer chronic depression, and many who have died by suicide, have been shown to have significantly elevated levels of glucocorticoids, cortisol and other stress chemicals in their blood and tissues.

The constant bombardment from stress chemicals potentially underlies many of the physical symptoms of depression. Weight gain, hypertension, suppressed immune system, heart problems, can all be attributed to the persistent action of stress chemicals in the body. All told, the claims that it's all in your head are starting to seem ever more dubious.

But speaking of your head, these stress chemicals and hormones seem to have a potent effect on neurons, and therefore the functioning of the brain. Specifically, they seem to

161

stimulate areas like the hippocampus and prefrontal cortex, to enhance our memory, and thinking, and focus. Because when you're in a stressful situation, you want to have your wits about you, and you don't want to forget what happens, because it could happen again, and you need to remember how to deal with it.

Unfortunately, this causes a problem. Neurons can handle a certain amount of increased signalling, of enhanced excitation. But too much leads to excitotoxicity, a phenomenon whereby excess activity damages, impairs, or sometimes even kills a neuron.[23] The complex biochemical processes a neuron engages in to do what it needs to do are quite demanding. Give them time to restock and replenish after pushing them to their limit, they'll be fine. But keep pushing them, and they'll suffer. Clog up. Break down. It's like trying to drive on the motorway with your car in second gear; your engine isn't going to last long. It's not meant to do that.

So, stress chemicals stimulate many areas of the brain. But when the HPA axis fails to stop pumping out the stress chemicals, those brain areas are stimulated too much, exhausting and damaging the neurons, causing them to lose plasticity. Simultaneously, there's no reason why other parts of the brain, with neurons that have subtly different properties, can't respond differently to the stress hormones, even be enhanced by them. To put it simply, there's a decent chance that it's the runaway stress response that causes all the issues of depression, inducing the physical symptoms, by constantly stimulating, and thus overworking, the neurons in certain key areas of the brain, and thus reducing neuroplasticity. Simultaneously, other important brain regions react differently and are enhanced by excess stress chemicals. to the extent that they become dominant, to a disruptive extent.[51]

The obvious example of the latter would be the amygdala, a part of the brain that is integral to our fear and aversion responses. A life of constant stress would need a more active amygdala, to keep on top of things. Unless the constant stress was a mistake: as in, the brain is producing a stress response where the circumstances technically don't warrant one. This does explain a lot of what we've covered about depression. The depleted neuroplasticity in certain regions explains numerous symptoms. An enhanced amygdala and heightened stress reaction would explain why it's so easy to relapse and fall back into a depressive episode, particularly in response to a stressful experience, as so many seem to do. The neuroplasticity of the affected regions may bounce back following therapies of whatever kind, but enhanced brain regions tend to linger if they're still being used. And when does life stop being stressful in any way, shape or form? If you have an enhanced stress response as it is, it doesn't take much more stress to start the process all over again.

It also helps explain why a constant, maintenance dose of antidepressants is a very helpful therapeutic strategy in many cases of depression. The persistent level of antidepressants may be cancelling out the increased power of the stress reaction in the brain, helping to keep it in check. It can also explain why cognitive behavioural therapy combined with antidepressants can be the most useful approach.

Rachel England has experienced this first-hand:

I regularly take antidepressants; they work for me. But I have also seen a lot of therapists in my time. One was an absolutely ancient, almost decrepit old man who was wearing a tweed jacket and stank of mothballs. I was just fifteen at the time. They parked me in this room with him and he just looked at my notes and said, 'Were you uh, were you born by caesarean?' I said yes. He said 'Aaah,' and at that point I thought right, screw this.

Then there was this woman therapist who very obviously subscribed to a lot of schools of Freudian thought. She was asking me all of these questions about my dad. Not the, 'Do you feel like you live up to his expectations?' kind of questions, but things like, 'Do you ever think about your father?' You know: 'You're fourteen, you are at an important age of your development.' I was just like, 'Oh God.' I'm a teenager but I know that that's gross. So, I'm leaving.

Years later, when I lived in London, I was attacked quite violently, and in the aftermath the police gave me a pamphlet: 'So, you've been a victim of violent crime. Do you want some therapy?' And I was like, 'Why not? It can't hurt, can it, and I've got a lot of stuff going on in my head, so maybe it will be useful.'

I went along and what was supposed to be four government-funded sessions of this therapy turned into thirty-six weeks because this woman wanted to write about me in her PhD. I don't know what came of that, but it was

*phenomenally helpful, and it's therapy in that form that
was something I would certainly consider returning to
because it's really hard and unpleasant, but ultimately it
did help a lot.*

Why exactly would talking therapy combined with antidepressants work better than either alone? Aren't they completely different approaches? Well, one possibility is that
antidepressants may ensure the affected neurons regrow
their lost connections, but cognitive behavioural therapies,
which are all about making you think and mentally process
stuff in helpful ways, help *shape* these new connections, in
the most useful and enduringly beneficial manner.

So, we have an explanation for depression. For some reason, the brain's chemical response to stress malfunctions,
meaning the stress response doesn't shut down. And of
course, when we're overly stressed, it means we're in a negative emotional mindset, or a low mood. But if our brain is
saturated with stress chemicals, it causes the neurons in key
brain regions to be overstimulated, wearing them out and
causing them to lose plasticity, while simultaneously enhancing the more stress-centric brain processes. The loss of
flexibility and adaptability the excessive stress causes means
the low-mood state essentially becomes stuck.

Antidepressants, and other interventions, whether they
involve direct electrical stimulation or cognitive talking
therapies, increase activity in certain parts of the brain's
network, and this hopefully spreads to the affected areas
and restores normal functioning. Although some of the

unhelpful changes are enduring, meaning an oversensitivity to future stressful experiences, which can trigger the whole process all over again.

That all adds up, right? But then, perhaps this is, once again, too straightforward an explanation? It certainly seems all neat and tidy, while making logical sense. But then so did the monoamine hypothesis, not too long ago. Look how that ended up.

There's still so much to consider

It can't be repeated enough, but if you're hoping for firm, concrete answers to how mental health problems work in the brain, then I'm going to disappoint you. I don't have any. But, in my defence, nobody does. Anyone who claims they know exactly what's happening to cause mental health issues is either worryingly naïve, or actively misleading you.*

There are many scientists and mental health experts who wouldn't agree with my explanation of depression in terms of stress and neuroplasticity. Some point to the more cognitive aspects, arguing that the physical elements of the brain are not as important as the mental processes that arise from them, and how we experience and perceive them. Others focus on more genetic or cellular aspects, coming up with alternative mechanisms to explain the observed disruptions in a depressed brain. And many of these can be very compelling (if you can decipher the dense scientific jargon).

---

* Which is also worrying.

There's also an interesting school of thought that argues that depression is an *evolved process*. Meaning, it's meant to happen. It's a useful thing.[24] The logic goes that when we were a species that lived in the wild, in the world of tooth and claw, an incredibly stressful or traumatising event would potentially do lasting damage to your body and mind, and you'd need time to recuperate from this. But in a world without houses and books and Wi-Fi, a world where you never know where your next meal is coming from, where danger and risk are a constant presence, the idea of sitting still and giving yourself time to convalesce is a fanciful one.

Unless, that is, you were in a state where you had no motivation or desire to do anything; where you didn't want to interact, where your demanding neurological processes were at a very low ebb so you didn't need as much energy or stimulation. Such a condition would be useful after you've undergone something particularly harrowing, right? And so, it's argued, we experience depression, because it was useful, back in more primitive times.

It's a nice theory, and explains why depression is so common. But you should always be wary when encountering evolutionary psychology theories like this. There are plenty of legitimate theories in this area, but they're often reverse-engineered, meaning an everyday trait leads to someone creating a scenario from the distant past where it would have been useful, and just going with it. Given the timescales involved, it's pretty much impossible to disprove that something affected us and shaped our evolution over several million years. And a lot of the time, these theories have a rather sinister ideological bent.

167

It's like how women can't read maps, because traditionally it was the men in primitive tribes who went and hunted, meaning they needed more navigational and spatial skills. You might have heard that theory. But you shouldn't have. Because it's not true. As far as I know, there's no compelling evidence to suggest a fundamental difference in male and female brains when it comes to navigation. Nonetheless, if you wanted to show that men were intellectually superior to women on a fundamental level, this would be a handy theory to peddle.

The overall point here is, there's a lot going on in the brain when depression happens. And even if we could pin it all on one root cause, like stress, there's just so much going on in a typical brain. You'd still expect a wide range of different expressions and symptoms and effects from person to person. Expecting something that affects the brain at the fundamental, cellular level to have the same effect every time in every different brain is like repeatedly dropping a bucket of ping-pong balls into a raging river and expecting them to end up at the exact same downstream location each time. Not going to happen. That's why there are so many different types of depression, so many different treatments, so many different ranges of effectiveness, and so on.

In truth, we still don't know for certain how the brain works, and what happens in it to cause depression. We're fairly certain it's something, and we have a decent range of candidates now. All this, coupled with constant advances in research, medicine, and so on, means there is ample reason to be hopeful.

But all things being equal, the stress idea seems to be a very compelling one. And not just for depression.

4: Anxiety

If there's one thing the modern human brain is undisputedly the best at, it's finding things to worry about. Simpler creatures may only experience worry and fear in response to more tangible threats – genuine hazards to life and limb. However, our big brains give us a much wider scope for concerns.

Can I afford my rent this month?

That twinge in my leg, or tightness in my chest, is that something serious?

Am I thin enough? Tall enough? Muscular enough? Pretty enough?

Am I going to get to the airport on time?

Am I on the right bus?

Is this relationship going anywhere, or are we staying together just because it's easier?

And on, and on.

When people say things like 'Stop worrying' or 'Be grateful for what you've got', that's a much bigger ask than such simple (and patronising) instructions can ever convey. Even though us modern first-world humans lead much safer and more comfortable lives than our ancestors ever dared dream of, our brains still work in the same fundamental ways as they have done for millennia. Basically, the human brain is constantly looking for things to worry about.

This might sound like a bad thing, but it's likely one of the secrets of humankind's success. Being proficient at anticipating, and therefore avoiding, dangers and threats is an excellent survival tactic for a species living in a dangerous environment, like our human ancestors were for most of our evolutionary history. But we've only really tamed our environment, made it safe, in the last few thousand years, which is like eleven seconds ago on an evolutionary scale. So, we still have these deeply ingrained parts of our brain constantly on the lookout for dangers and threats. They've kept us alive for millions of years, after all.

Of course, in that time, we've also developed powerful intellects, brain regions and processes that can comprehend and retain and extrapolate information like never before. And these brain regions are linked to every other part, to a greater or lesser degree. As a result, we have these instinctive neurological processes, constantly monitoring for threats and hazards, married to the powerful intellectual parts, which can extrapolate and predict and anticipate. This means the human brain can anticipate and predict unpleasant or harmful events, then relay this information to the processes that respond to threats, meaning we can react to dangers *before they happen.*

In a nutshell, our brains are constantly looking for things to worry about. And because they can understand and recognise all the unpleasant things that can happen in our increasingly complicated world, we pretty much always find them. There's even the psychological phenomenon termed counterfactual thinking,[1] where people spend a lot of time worrying about alternative outcomes to past events, the 'what ifs' . . .

You've probably done it yourself.

What if that car that narrowly missed me . . . had actually hit me?

What if I'd given a different answer to that interview question and actually got the job?

What if I'd gone on that date instead of meeting with friends? I could be married to someone else now.

What if I'd been able to afford that holiday I wanted? I might have been there when the earthquake happened.

All of these are concerns based on something that didn't happen, and logically can*not* happen, because it's in the past. Yet do people still spend time worrying about them anyway? Absolutely. So, the human brain tends to worry. A lot. Way more than is useful. And this can cause us serious problems.

Another word for worries? Anxieties. It's normal, even healthy, for people to worry, to experience anxiety, in response to the challenges and issues they encounter in their lives. But for certain people, this anxiety becomes constant, excessive, illogical, and difficult, even impossible, to control. And that's when you get anxiety as a mental health problem, not just an everyday occurrence that's common to everyone.

There's a similar problem here to what we saw with depression earlier. Specifically, the term anxiety can mean either just generally worrying about something, or a serious and life-altering mental health issue. And this is not the only thing anxiety and depression have in common – trust me on this.

Regardless of terminology, anxiety is a major mental health problem. According to available data, it comes second only to depression with regards to the most common mental health problems worldwide,[2] although anxiety is perhaps more diverse than depression in terms of how it can manifest – so much so that what is or isn't an official anxiety disorder is constantly being reassessed and debated. We'll look at the diverse range of expression of anxiety later. But first, let's look at some of the basics of anxiety in the brain. What it is. What it's for. Where it comes from. Stuff like that.

The pros and cons of anxiety

We've established that the human brain is an intensely cautious organ, having evolved many dedicated systems and processes that keep us aware of, and responsive to, threats and dangers. Many scientists refer to this as the threat detection system, so that's what I'm going to call it here.

Importantly, this threat detection system isn't passive; it doesn't just sit there and flag up hazards but then do nothing about them, like an utterly apathetic security guard. No, when the threat detection system spots something that is, or could be, dangerous, it gets stuck right in. It puts out multiple chemical and neurological signals that make us alert and ready our body and brain to deal with the recognised threat.

This is the fight-or-flight response in action again: we become primed to tackle the danger or problem, or get away from it. But it's not an all or nothing thing – and that's important. True, the threat detection system does seem to be very sensitive, maintaining constant vigilance, and with something of a hair trigger. But it also takes into account the severity, type or nature of the threat. All these things dictate how substantial our reaction is. Because we can't just run screaming at, or away from, literally everything that gives us reason to worry.

For instance, some studies show that the threat detection system shows raised activity in response to basic triangles.[3] Yes, there's evidence to suggest we're instinctively afraid of *triangles*. Sounds ridiculous, I know, but consider that these threat detection systems evolved over millions of years, out in the wild. What sort of things would be dangerous there? Predators, with their sharp teeth, or talons, or claws, or beaks? Spiky plants? Jagged rocks to fall into? A lot of dangerous things in nature are basically triangular. Pointy. So, an instinctive wariness of such things would be a useful survival trait, and one we seem to still possess today.

173

But obviously, triangles activate our threat detection systems only mildly. We don't run screaming at the sight of a wizard's hat, or furiously launch ourselves at anyone holding a slice of pizza. It's more of a sliding scale; minor threats provoke more of a 'keep an eye on that for now' response, whereas severe dangers right in front of you set off all the alarm bells, get the heart racing, the panic surging, and so on. And there's everything in between.

I know I explained this earlier, but it warrants repeating: the stress response is seemingly due to the brain's threat detection system preparing us to deal with dangers and threats. It's the precursor to the fear, the fight-or-flight response. It's like the build-up to the main event, the minions in a video game that you deal with before the big boss battle.

And while the feeling of stress and anxiety is subjectively unpleasant, it's usually a good thing. The sort of thing that keeps us safe, unharmed, and, in some cases, alive. It's not just about keeping us safe, either – have you heard about people who thrive under pressure? Apparently, we all do that, to an extent. Because unlike being depressed, being anxious and stressed puts you in an active state. It makes you *aroused*.*

The stress response increases muscle tension, raises heart and breathing rate, makes you more focused, less distractable, and more motivated. For most jobs – be they factory-floor worker, professional athlete or astronaut – this state makes you better able to fulfil your duties. Countless studies have

---

* To clarify, that's aroused in the scientific sense, of being in a heightened, energetic state. Not 'sexy fun times' aroused. Although it depends on what you're into, I guess?

shown that, up to a point, a person's performance increases directly in proportion to how much stress they're experiencing. But the key phrase here is 'up to a point'. Because eventually, stress becomes a hindrance, and further increasing stress makes performance worse.

If you show this on a graph where performance is plotted against experience of stress, it turns into a very neat curve, like an upside-down U, where performance goes up as you increase stress, reaches a peak, and falls right back down again if stress keeps increasing. This graph is called the Yerkes-Dodson curve, just so you know.[4]

The comparison I like to use is salt. No salt in your food, it's bland and unpalatable. Add salt, and it tastes increasingly good. But at some point, it becomes too much salt. Your food goes from increasingly tasty to an intense, gritty, heart-clogging ordeal. Continuing to add salt just makes it worse.

The thing is, becoming more aroused and tense and focused when dealing with an immediate issue may be a good thing, but being constantly primed for danger, over long periods, is demanding, draining and disruptive. A smoke alarm going off when there's actual smoke to deal with is helpful. A smoke alarm going off constantly is infuriating, and wears out the battery and workings much faster. Lord help you if there's an actual fire to deal with.

Thankfully, our brains have systems in place to keep the threat detection system under control, to make sure it doesn't run amok, to shut it down again when it's not needed. Unfortunately, it seems that for those with an anxiety disorder, these neurological systems stop working, so the threat response keeps running when it's not meant to. You remain on high alert, constantly looking for – and primed to respond to – dangers, threats and hazards. Again, that's basically what stress is. And it takes its toll, on our bodies and brains.

This admittedly sounds very similar to much of what was just said about the mechanisms underlying depression. The last chapter went into great detail about how the HPA axis, that neurological circuit that governs the physical and chemical response to stress, stops regulating itself and keeps pumping out the stress substances, leading to depression. Isn't that another way of saying 'a threat response that doesn't shut down'? It's a valid point. The truth is, the same uninhibited-stress process is increasingly believed to underlie depression *and* anxiety. We'll look more closely at how and why later.

But first, to briefly summarise, anxiety, meaning the mental health disorder, is widely believed to be down to what's called a disinhibition of the threat detection and response system. In even simpler terms, there are parts of the brain that cause us to experience fear, worry and stress whenever we encounter problems and hazards, and there are other parts of the brain responsible for shutting them down when required. Anxiety is what happens when those latter parts of the brain are no longer effective.

That's an undeniably simple description of what's going on, and while it's pretty much an accurate one, it doesn't come close to conveying just how vastly complicated this whole system is. So, which bit of the brain is doing what? And where do the problems arise?

The all-powerful amygdala

The threat detection system isn't a single, discrete thing. There are many brain regions involved in simply recognising that something may be a threat. You've got all the sensory information and the systems that process it letting us know all the things going on around and inside us, any one of which could prove threatening. There are also all the internal cognitive processes, all the thoughts and rationalisations and imagination that allow us to anticipate and recognise possible threats to our well-being, or our situation, because we humans aren't limited to experiencing fear and anxiety purely in response to real, physical dangers to life and limb.

So, great swathes of the brain are involved in recognising and responding to threats, which unfortunately makes anxiety a very variable and stubborn problem to pin down and deal with. But it's not completely befuddling, because there seem to be a few key brain areas involved.

Some of them are more fundamental, long-established areas, buried deeper in the midbrain. These are the areas that deal with the more primitive, instinctive stuff, as you might expect. On top of this, though, there are many advanced brain regions involved in threat detection and reactions, located in the more recently evolved neocortex: the big wrinkly bit on top of the brain. Those in the frontal lobe in particular have important roles in how we deal with threats and concerns.

To clarify, the brain has several layers, from neocortex on top, to midbrain underneath that, with brainstem and associated regions at the bottom. In a way, it's a bit like the rings in the trunk of a tree, with layer after layer being added as the tree gets older and larger. That comparison is particularly useful here because, as a general rule, the higher something is in the brain (as in, the closer to the outer surface), the more recently evolved it is. And the more recently evolved a brain area is, the more complex and advanced it tends to be, and the more sophisticated are the functions it handles. The most sophisticated part of the brain, the neocortex, appeared in our species over the past two million years or so. In comparison, the more fundamental parts of the brain, like those in the midbrain, have been around for at least ten times as long. For certain parts of the brain, like the brainstem, it's substantially longer again. We're talking about the dinosaur era, here.*

The prefrontal cortex, right behind your forehead, is the most advanced bit of the brain. Most of the difficult, abstract, conscious stuff stems from here: your sense of self, rational thought, critical and analytical thinking, and so on.

The main function of the higher brain regions, in the context of anxiety and stress, seems to be controlling, or modulating, emotions and worries. You could say they interpret and decipher the raw data that are generated by fear and other emotional reactions. This makes sense, as such higher brain regions are normally concerned with complex, conscious processes. The ones that allow us self-control, the ability to think for ourselves. This is often referred to as executive functioning.

* Hence the term 'the reptile brain'.

178

Meanwhile, the deeper, older parts of the brain generate the actual emotions, reflexes and immediate responses – things we experience without having to think about it. So, the visceral, subconscious fear response, the one that underpins so much anxiety and stress, almost certainly emerges from here.

There are several key brain regions at work.

There's the hippocampus, mainly responsible for memory processing, which allows us to learn what is and isn't a threat and respond accordingly.

There's the anterior cingulate cortex, which has multiple roles, including recognising negative social events and causing psychological pain, which helps explain why humans are so sensitive to social anxiety and embarrassment (as we'll soon see).

There's the periaqueductal grey, a small but versatile region, again with many functions, one of which is triggering our defensive reactions when deemed necessary, like tensing up, breathing and heart rate becoming more rapid, and so on.

But if there's one part of the brain that's been the central focus of anxiety research for as long as it's been happening, it would be the amygdala.

The amygdala was mentioned a lot in the previous chapter on depression, for good reason. To reiterate, it's a relatively small, almond-shaped nucleus, which has multiple, crucial roles, most of which are emotional in nature.[5] The amygdala adds the emotional element of memories, allowing us to recall and re-experience how we felt at the time, not just what happened. There's evidence to suggest it also determines what emotional reaction is required in any given situation.[6]

If someone takes all their clothes off in front of you, should you become sexually aroused? If it's your romantic partner in your bedroom, then yes, that would, presumably, be an appropriate reaction. If it's a stranger in the gym changing-room, or someone you're about to perform a cavity search on, then no, definitely not. The same act can lead to very different responses in your brain. And it's believed to be the amygdala that determines this. It weighs up all the available data, considers the situation, and decides what reaction is warranted.

The amygdala is central to the emotion processing regions of the midbrain, commonly known as the limbic system. Ergo, the amygdala and emotional reactions go hand in hand. But still, the most well-known and well-established role of the amygdala is the fear response. While many parts of the brain are involved in recognising and responding to threats, it's the amygdala that has the most clout here. It's the part of the brain that says, 'Yes, this particular thing warrants worrying about, so prep the body and mind for high alert.' And so, we get the stress response, or the fear response, or the panic response, depending on how threatening the thing is. A judgement made, it seems, by the amygdala.

Given all it does, the amygdala has a very wide range of complex, detailed connections with many other parts of the brain. These connections run to both the higher brain regions, like the prefrontal cortex, which handles things like thinking and self-control, and the lower regions, like the

HPA axis, which induces the physical stress response via release of numerous hormones.

For a long time, it was assumed that anxiety disorders were down to the amygdala being overly active. If activity in the amygdala is responsible for creating worry and anxiousness, then it follows that too much activity will result in too much anxiety being experienced. Makes sense. And mostly, this argument holds up. Amygdala hyperactivity is observed in countless anxiety studies,[7] and anything that lowers activity in the amygdala invariably reduces signs of fear, distress and, yes, anxiety.

But, as ever, it's more complex than that. As central as it may be to the brain's processing of fear and worry, the amygdala doesn't exist in isolation. There are many brain regions that control, guide or limit its effects, where necessary. Or, at least, they should do that.

What are these regions, and why do they sometimes not do their jobs?

The smart, rational prefrontal cortex

I stated earlier that humans are better at worrying than most other species, because our brains are smart enough to recognise a much wider range of things that might negatively affect us. Do rats worry about losing their job? Does a pigeon get stressed when trying to outbid someone on an eBay auction? Are sheep kept awake at night by gloomy economic forecasts? No. They aren't aware of the existence of such things.

This isn't to say these species have easier lives than us, but the risks and dangers that stress them out are more tangible, more 'real', than much of what stresses us out. Presumably, this means that simpler creatures rely on simpler ways of shutting down the fear and stress response, like the chemical feedback effect of the HPA axis covered earlier. In the harsh world of nature, a threat is typically one that either kills you or goes away. If it goes away, those threat-detecting regions of animal brains no longer detect the threat, so stop sounding the alarm. Or the brain, along with the rest of the animal, is dead.

Either way, the fear response stops.

Obviously, this isn't so easy with the human brain. The trouble is, the amygdala and other aspects of the threat detection system react in the same way, whether we're venturing down a dark alley in a crime-ridden area or giving a presentation at work. The size or extent of the response can differ, but our fundamental reactions to a threat are essentially fixed. Our brains just don't discriminate that well between genuine physical hazards right in front of us and abstract unpleasant occurrences that may happen in our future.

Basically, the threat detection system only has a limited range of responses to perceived dangers, and it uses them like an emergency horn. You can adjust the volume, sound it frequently or rarely, but it's still the same noise that's played. This causes problems because, again, we humans constantly fret about things that might happen, or things that didn't happen, but could have. And we worry about things like self-image, or how other people perceive us, or our long-term goals. These things are hugely subjective and very speculative, so often can't manifest in the real world in any useful, tangible way.

And here's the problem: it's very difficult to know if, or when, we can stop being anxious about these things. If we're worrying about things that haven't happened, when do we stop worrying? How can a threat be recognised as 'gone away' when it was technically never there to begin with?

It's a recipe for a constant, never-ending stress response. And it shows how tricky, and slippery, control of the stress and anxiety response can be in the hugely complex human brain. Thankfully, among the many sophisticated processes our brain has evolved, there are also more advanced means of controlling or limiting the output of the amygdala, thus curbing our reactions to fear and stress. And if there's any bit of the brain that you'd expect to be tackling the vivid, instinctive, emotional output of the amygdala, it's the prefrontal cortex, responsible for self-control, analysis, rational thought, inhibitions, and so on.

And that's pretty much exactly what happens.

But, as ever, the relationship between the prefrontal cortex and the amygdala is not straightforward. The prefrontal cortex doesn't just stop the amygdala when it goes too far, like a teacher breaking up a fight in a school playground, or someone playing whack-a-mole. Interestingly, while the prefrontal cortex and amygdala regularly oppose each other, they also frequently cooperate. They exchange much information, work together, and affect each other in many complex ways. It's sort of like a marriage in a classic sitcom; endless bickering and arguing, but they're still committed to each other.

The prefrontal cortex is also believed to be the part that makes sense of all the confusing and complex information sloshing around in our brains. It's the part that translates it all into something coherent, something useful, that we can perceive and think about. Like how your laptop or tablet takes raw binary code coming in from your broadband cable and turns it into Netflix shows and cat memes. While it's the amygdala that's responsible for the underlying fear response, it's arguably the prefrontal cortex that translates it into feelings of anxiety.

It's also important to remember that this connection isn't one-way. The prefrontal cortex seems crucial for all our calculation and deduction and forward planning. Therefore, it's what works out intangible, potential threats and dangers, like possible embarrassment, a relationship breakdown, or losing a job. This information, about these potential threats and hazards, is shared with the amygdala, which triggers the fear response, which makes us anxious.

As well as this, the amygdala and prefrontal cortex can operate independently of each other. Have you ever been alone at home, sitting quietly by yourself, then heard something smash? It's frightening. You're suddenly scared, tense, your heart is hammering, you've got gooseflesh, and so on. It's a very normal reaction. Usually, once you stop and think about it, you quickly figure out there's nothing to fear. That smash was probably that picture falling off the wall. The wobbly one, that you've been telling your partner to fix or take down for weeks.

But even though you work out that there's nothing to worry about, you still experienced a fear response. If something unexpected and jarring happens, your threat detection system jumps into action right away. Sensory information gets fed to your amygdala without the conscious brain's involvement, and when something like that occurs, it instantly sounds the alarm, regardless of whether you think it's warranted. It's because this emotional reaction is older and simpler than our ability to consciously think something through logically, which means it's a lot faster too. You don't even have time to consider whether it's valid. You don't have time to *consider*, full stop.

Higher parts of the brain, like the prefrontal cortex, simply can't keep up with these ancient hardwired reflexes and emotions, but what they *can* do is limit your emotional reaction, or modulate it. It's like a human walking a dog on a lead. A big, powerful dog, like a St Bernard. The person can guide the dog, issue commands, and pull on the lead if needs be. But they can't control what the dog is thinking or doing. They're mostly limited to reacting to what it does, like paying for breakages, or apologising to anyone it's jumped up and slobbered on. And the dog, as big as it is, may well break free of the lead, and bound around doing its own thing.

In this analogy, the person is the prefrontal cortex, and the dog is the amygdala, or the emotional system in general. The person is smarter, sure, but that doesn't necessarily mean they have total control. And when the dog escapes from the lead? And the person is running flat out after it, desperately trying to catch it and stop it causing chaos? That's anxiety.

Prefrontal vs amygdala, in the fight for anxiety

Why, though? Why does the prefrontal cortex (and associated regions) lose control? How does the amygdala end up being so dominant? There are multiple factors at work here, but an important one is that the balance between the amygdala and the prefrontal cortex – between fear, worry and anxiety, and rational thought and logic – is always in flux. It's not fixed or locked in. It makes sense that balance between the emotional, impulsive parts of the brain and the rational, self-control parts would be quasi-stable, at most. There are plenty of times when a fearful, anxious reaction is entirely appropriate. And there are times when it would be seriously unhelpful. Different situations call for different reactions. Remember what I said earlier: laughing aloud at a best man's speech is appropriate. Laughing at a eulogy is not.

If the brain were fixed so that either the emotional or the rational system always took priority, there would be many times when we'd react inappropriately, or too slowly, to unpredicted events. But while useful, this complex balance between the two systems is also fragile. It can be easily disrupted, or thrown out of whack, hence anxiety disorders are as common as they are. This is especially clear during adolescence, a period of our lives when the brain rapidly starts maturing, clearing away the clutter of childhood, and making everything more efficient, to prepare for adult life. But here's the issue: the simpler a brain region is, the less time it takes to mature. And the amygdala and limbic systems are older, therefore simpler, parts of the brain. They don't take long to mature, so reach peak efficiency early on in adolescence.

By contrast, the prefrontal cortex and associated regions are the most complex parts of the brain, and evidence suggests they aren't fully mature until we're around twenty-five! So, throughout our teens, our emotional systems are working at maximum efficiency, while our prefrontal regions, which keep emotions in line via restraint and control, are still a work in progress, struggling to keep up. Hence, your teenage years are when you're at your most emotional. It's not that teens can't control their emotions, it's just that doing so requires more effort, at a time when their emotions are more potent than they've ever been.

Basically, during early adolescence, the amygdala has the upper hand more often, so the emotional reactions produced by the amygdala, particularly fear and worry, are more prominent. Do you remember being a teen? Remember how every social interaction seemed so nerve-wracking? How everything was a drama, how everything made you intensely angry or miserable? How the very thought of asking someone out could make you hyperventilate? How any rejection felt like the end of the world? Doesn't that sound like what would happen in a brain where the emotional systems are more dominant than they should be?

There are also interesting data that show that anxiety is a considerable issue with adolescent mental health, but is more common during the earlier years – say, ages eleven to thirteen – and gradually declines into late teens.[8] One explanation is that, earlier on, the newly matured amygdala and associated

187

threat detection system have the most sway, so keep things on high alert, meaning young teens are way more nervous about way more things. But as they grow and learn, the prefrontal cortex and other self-control systems become better able to keep the emotional systems in check. They figure out that intense, panic-inducing fear is a disproportionate response to saying hello to someone attractive, so override the amygdala when it tries to react like this. And the stronger and more mature the prefrontal cortex gets, the better able it is to counteract the immediate, anxiety-inducing emotional impulses that are particularly prominent in early teens.

That's one theory anyway. There's a lot going on in the developing brain, so there are undoubtedly multiple factors at work. But hopefully this helps you understand what it's like when the threat and emotional response processes in the brain have more impact than the rational, self-control ones. It's something we all experienced during our earlier years, and some of you may be going through it right now. And hopefully it helps us to appreciate that there are plenty of times in our lives when we *should* let our emotions guide us, because that's the right thing to do. Times of urgency, times of grief, in intimate relationships. There are times when a cold, rational analysis just doesn't help, or can actively make things worse.

However, when the balance shifts too far one way – when the amygdala and the threat detection systems wield too much influence over our thoughts and feelings, and our rational processes struggle or fail to regain the upper hand – that's when we get serious anxiety.

As always, multiple brain parts and processes play a role in anxiety. Accordingly, clinical anxiety can be expressed in a variety of ways.

Let's look at some of those.

Generalised anxiety disorder, and the clinical side of anxiety

In 2017, the World Health Organization estimated that 264 million people worldwide were living with anxiety disorders. And that number's seemingly only going up. Meanwhile, depression cases numbered 322 million, making it still the more common disorder overall.[9]

That said, one interesting point to note is that some data suggest anxiety is more common than depression in the US specifically.[10] Some estimates suggest 40 million Americans are affected by anxiety each year. Other estimates peg it even higher, with one in five of the population of the US experiencing anxiety disorders.

Why would the American population be more anxious overall? Is there some unique trait of the American psyche that makes people more prone to anxiety? Or is there something in American culture that puts people more on edge, gives them more to worry about? I'm sure we can all speculate and argue about that for quite some time, but it's beyond my remit here.

It's worth flagging up, though, that this is unlikely to be a specific quirk of the American brain. Remember in Chapter 1, where we talked about how mental health issues are often determined by comparing someone's thinking and behaviour to established cultural norms? This can be an issue, because the norms of a culture can and do change over time. But these norms also undeniably differ *between* cultures. One culture will think differently about important matters, compared to another. That's basically *why* they're considered different cultures! Wouldn't it logically follow, then, that the expression and assessment of mental health problems would also differ? Technically, yes it would. And it does.

For instance, the fields of social psychology and sociology have long noted that Western cultures tend to be more individualistic, meaning self-worth and self-fulfilment is the main goal for most. Eastern cultures, on the other hand, lean more towards collectivism, where the community, or family, or cultural traditions take priority. This is, admittedly, a very broad generalisation, and it's not that one approach is better than the other; both have their pros and cons. My point is, if your brain develops in a certain cultural context, then it'll absorb the norms and understandings of that culture, which shapes how we think, act, and perceive things.

One result of this is, if someone starts thinking and behaving in ways that aren't in keeping with the culture they're a part of, they could be deemed as mentally abnormal, whereas in another culture they'd still be considered perfectly typical.

Earlier we discussed how, until relatively recently, it was the expert consensus in Western culture that homosexuality was a mental disorder. By contrast, the ancient Greeks, nearly 3,000 years ago, seemingly didn't even *have* a concept of a specific sexual orientation.[11] So, anyone being attracted to members of the same sex then wouldn't have warranted a raised eyebrow, let alone a diagnosis.*

This cultural variation in social norms and behaviours is one reason why people object to the DSM being so widely used; it's the creation of the American Psychiatric Association, composed primarily of individuals who grew up, live, trained and practise in America, a very affluent first-world nation. How are their conclusions about what is and isn't normal behaviour and thinking relevant to a teenager living in the rural areas of Botswana, or a retiree in the heart of Shanghai?

As an aside, that's another good reason why I like to focus on the brain. While each individual brain is unique overall, there are still plenty of gross structures and properties that all brains have in common, and this can give some consistency to mental health matters, even though the ultimate expression of them may differ considerably from individual to individual.

To put this in simpler terms, everyone may have a different type of brain that can go wrong in its own special way due to who they are, how their life goes, and what culture they belong to. But everyone begins with essentially the same basic brain starter pack, so they all run on similar systems at the more fundamental levels.

Predictably, this cultural differentiation regarding mental health makes studying it even more frustrating. Just now, I gave the worldwide occurrences of depression and anxiety,

---

* Some modern conservative types might argue that this means the entire ancient Greek culture was mentally unwell, but they sure got a lot done if that was the case.

useful numbers to be aware of – but figures like these should still be approached warily, because mental health issues and problems can be hard to pin down.

One reason for this, which both feeds into and is compounded by the fact that diagnosis is not an exact science, is that mental health issues can manifest in very different ways, from person to person, as well as culture to culture. Is a case of depression in the heart of Tibet the same as one in the suburbs of Chicago? Presumably not. But will two cases of depression in Tibet be the exact same? Again, probably not.

Let's bring this diversion back to the subject at hand, namely anxiety, and how it works. While these cultural and individual variations hinder the establishing of a thorough and reliable understanding of mental health problems in general, they seem particularly irksome when it comes to the anxiety disorders in particular, as anxiety is one of the more variable conditions.

Let's start with the basics. For most, anxiety suggests being perpetually worried, stressed, nervous, 'strung out', to an incapacitating degree, and maybe for no discernible reason. In this case, they're probably thinking of generalised anxiety disorder, GAD. It's essentially the figurehead of anxiety disorders, in that it's the one people usually picture when they think of anxiety, just as major depressive disorder occupies that role for depression. As usual, according to the psychiatric approach, there are certain criteria that must be present before a diagnosis of generalised anxiety disorder can be made. And as ever, there are many who dispute these criteria, saying they're too narrow or too rigid to truly reflect what an individual is experiencing.

I know I keep highlighting this, but it's important. In the case of anxiety, the focus on someone being persistently worried or stressed out is often deemed too narrow, or too specific. Many report anxiety disorders that are expressed via constant anger or irritability rather than stress and worry. But for now, I'm going to focus on the more familiar expression, of literal anxiety.

The criteria for generalised anxiety disorder are, helpfully, roughly the same in both the DSM and ICD.[12] The primary element of generalised anxiety disorder is excessive anxiety and worry, on most days, in response to everyday events and problems. It's not that someone is constantly worried about things that *do* warrant a degree of concern or apprehension; it's that they're excessively worried about numerous things (hence the term generalised) to an extent that's not rational or proportional. It's fine to be worried about things like work deadlines or imminent weddings. But if you're *so* worried you can't even function or think straight, then there's cause for concern.

More parallels can be drawn with depression here – it's fine to be sad or depressed when a situation warrants it, but it's when you're excessively, persistently depressed for no obvious reason that something may be up with your mental health.

Both the DSM and ICD stipulate that generalised anxiety disorder also comes with numerous physical symptoms, such as accelerated heart rate, sweating, trembling or shaking, dry mouth, and more. There can also be chest pains, nausea, numbness, hot flushes and/or chills, muscle tension, difficulty breathing, and so on. Generalised anxiety disorder is very generous with the physical consequences.

There are other cognitive issues too: irritability, difficulty focusing, or having your mind just go blank, disrupted sleep and being easily fatigued, restlessness, or 'feeling on edge', as the kids say. And those experiencing the anxiety, in whatever form it takes, *can't stop it*, even though they're usually aware that it's not logical, that it's a disproportionate response to what's actually happening. You know how certain people insist on telling those with depression to cheer up, as if it's that simple, and something they've not thought of? Well, telling someone with generalised anxiety disorder to 'chill out' or 'stop worrying' is similarly unhelpful. And patronising. They would stop worrying if they could, but they can't! That's why it's a clinical problem.

As mentioned, generalised anxiety disorder has many aspects in common with depressive disorders. Both are essentially an extreme and inflexible expression of an otherwise normal emotional, or cognitive, state. Both include many physical symptoms, despite famously being mental health issues, which again emphasises how limited such simple binary distinctions can be. Also, one of the main types of medication for anxiety is SSRIs – antidepressants. Does this mean there's a common cause that links both disorders? Possibly, yes.

However, there are important ways in which depression and anxiety differ. Remember how for a diagnosis of major depressive disorder, the key symptoms, such as severely

194

low mood, must be present for at least two weeks? In contrast, the symptoms for generalised anxiety disorder must be present for *six months* before a diagnosis is made. While many argue that this is excessive, for good reasons, there is an underlying logic to it.

Just now, I went into great detail (again) about how mental health problems are often recognised based on how much a person's thinking and behaviour differ from what's deemed normal by the society or culture in which they live. Well, in first-world nations it's relatively rare for someone who's mentally healthy to find themselves stuck in a low-mood, zero-motivation state. The average person's mood changes rapidly, and often, so a severely negative one persisting for two whole weeks is already concerning.

That's not true for anxiety, though. Someone with fine mental health could well be constantly worrying about something, or several somethings, for weeks, even months, on end. Big project at work? Planning a wedding? Having a baby? Buying a house? These are common occurrences, but also significant, long-lasting commitments, with ample opportunities for something to go wrong, and thus regularly cause intense and prolonged anxiety and worry.

But this anxiety is, for want of a better word, normal. A logical response to what's happening. Ergo, not a problem, per se. And there we can see why it's difficult to separate generalised anxiety disorder from regular everyday anxiety. Only when it keeps happening, over an excessively long period, can we be sure that there's something going on that *shouldn't* be happening.

The different culture aspect of mental health comes up quite often here. I've been asked many times about whether people in more primitive cultures, such as those in remote tribes, are happier than we in the developed world are. Is there something to be said for a simpler existence? Personally, I'd argue that this is a huge oversimplification, and that those who 'live off the land' and whatnot have other types of issues and stresses that we're blissfully unaware of.

But it could reasonably be said that our 'developed society' lives are more complex, and therefore have more things that stress us out, because there's just a lot more going on in our world. And remember, the parts of our brain that handle threat and stress don't discern between genuinely life-endangering hazards and intangible, abstract dangers, like job loss or embarrassment.

It could be that those who live in less complex societies experience greater, life-endangering stresses, but more rarely, while those of us in first-world cultures have a more constant, background sort of stress, and therefore anxiety, which can sometimes prove overwhelming to our brain's system, leading to generalised anxiety disorder.

But this isn't to say that anxiety can't overwhelm us in one intense burst.

Attacks of panic

Another type of anxiety disorder is panic disorder, a particularly potent issue where someone experiences regular panic attacks. Generalised anxiety disorder, with all its myriad symptoms, is regularly debilitating, but in a more gradual way. The afflicted person is worn down with the perpetual stress and disruption caused by constant anxiety. Panic attacks, in contrast, involve a lot of the same symptoms, such as pounding and rapid heart rate, trembling, shaking, sweating, dry mouth, sickness, chest pain and dizziness, but they hit you all at once, in one intense burst.

If the symptoms of anxiety were like getting wet, generalised anxiety disorder is akin to being caught in a persistent downpour, while panic attacks are like getting hit with a high-pressure fire hose; as well as being left shaking and soaked, you're also knocked off your feet, and left floundering for several minutes.

Here's Girl on the Net, with her own personal experience of such a thing . . .

The worst time I had a panic attack was when I got trapped at Stratford Westfield, where they've now got West Ham football club inside the Olympic Stadium. I went to go and meet someone there and go on the big slide, which you used to be able to do out of one of the towers near the stadium.

So I had all this adrenaline from doing the big slide, and then I walked out just as the football crowd was kicking out – and I panicked. I had to walk through this football crowd, and I had a panic attack right in the middle of this huge group of chanting football men.

I feel awful about it because at least two or three nice football men came up to me and were like, 'You all right love?' But I couldn't breathe and I couldn't say anything,

> *and I was crying and panicky, so was just like 'Fuck off,*
> *just fuck off,' and then had to go and sit by the side of the*
> *road and just try and escape while everybody walked past*
> *me. It was this horrible sea of people.*
>
> *Now I'm much better at just escaping the situation. I've*
> *done quite a lot of talking therapy to get to that point. So,*
> *as long as I'm not trapped in a situation, I feel comfortable*
> *and I can deal with whatever's coming.*

One (very minor) positive is that panic attacks, while very intense, are relatively short-lived. Typically, a genuine panic attack builds up, peaks, and ebbs away in a matter of minutes.[13] They're still incredibly awful, but we're not talking about something that goes on for days on end.

However, a diagnosis of panic disorder isn't limited to experiencing attacks. The DSM states that there should be at least one month of persistent worry and concerns about having an attack.

Or, persistent changes in behaviour related to the attacks – as in, people behave differently because they're constantly preoccupied with the possibility of having an attack.

Or, persistent worry about what an attack means: is it a symptom of some deep-rooted and serious health problem they weren't aware of? Things like that.

One, all, or a combination of these features is necessary for a diagnosis of panic disorder, according to the DSM.

However, one intriguing aspect of panic attacks is that there's often no obvious cause, or trigger event.[14] There *can* be events or triggers that set them off, sure. But just as often, if not more so, there isn't one. Of course, given how much the average person is experiencing at any given moment, it could be that there *is* a trigger for every attack, but one that isn't clear or recognisable, so can't be identified – but either way, it amounts to the same thing in practical terms, i.e. avoiding the cause of panic attacks is not an option.

Overall, then, there's often no recognisable pattern regarding how and when panic attacks occur, which tends to make people even more stressed, more anxious. The human brain is stressed out by unpredictable things as it is, because things being unpredictable and uncertain prevents us from anticipating and dealing with them on our own terms – it robs us of control. An unpredictable *threat* is worse again. That's the ideal thing for raising activity in the threat detection system, and when that's already ramped up, as it is in an anxiety disorder, it just makes everything worse. No wonder someone with panic disorder is constantly preoccupied by the attacks – when there's no way to anticipate them, why *wouldn't* you be constantly braced for them?

However, there are some anxiety disorders that do have definite, blatant triggers, or causes. And they're hardly any easier to deal with.

The endurance of PTSD

Post-traumatic stress disorder, aka PTSD, is a condition whereby someone experiences an event so terrible that it seriously disrupts their mental health afterwards. The impact of the event is too great to process and deal with normally.

More specifically, it's the experience of an event that involves serious threats to safety and/or bodily integrity, either to themselves, or to someone else. In the latter case, the person – while not directly involved – witnesses the event, and is unable to act. Basically, highly stimulating events that involve intense feelings of danger, horror, violation or helplessness, or any combination of these things, such as observing a hideous car crash, can lead to PTSD.

However, it's not just the experiencing of the event that leads to PTSD – not everyone who has deeply unpleasant experiences develops PTSD. Think of people in the emergency services, such as firefighters and paramedics, who deal with horrible events and situations as part of their job. Many of them seem able to keep going in spite of these stresses, perhaps protected by their training and their ability to intervene and act. In any case, others struggle to cope with what an objective observer may consider to be a lesser calamity, or event, and develop PTSD where other people wouldn't. But, as ever, it's not always so straightforward.

For example, someone who is homeless has undoubtedly experienced more unpleasant events than someone wealthy, living in a mansion. Therefore, you'd expect the former to be more likely to develop PTSD. And, in general, you'd probably be right.

On the other hand, living on the streets needn't be the result of one traumatic incident, but multiple, gradual misfortunes. While still awful, this is less likely to result in PTSD. But if the mansion owner ended up watching it, and everything in it, be destroyed by fire, having only just got out alive, that would be deeply traumatic. Traumatic enough to result in PTSD? Maybe.

The person living on the streets undoubtedly has a much worse life overall, but it could still be the rich person with the gutted home who develops PTSD. Anyway, it's what happens *after* a traumatic event that defines PTSD, that fulfils the criteria for a diagnosis.

PTSD is often associated with memories of the event that are incredibly vivid, and persistent.[15] People keep recalling specific aspects of the trauma, in painful detail. Or, they keep dreaming about it. Or, become severely anxious when encountering anything that reminds them of the experience, however indirectly. Or any combination of these things.

Such things are undeniably debilitating – so much so that those with PTSD often practise avoidance behaviour, where they actively, or even unknowingly, avoid anything they associate with the traumatic event. For example, if your trauma involved a car crash, you might then desperately avoid anything that involves cars. And how much of modern life involves car travel? A ridiculous amount.

Thanks to the vivid and persistent recall of the event, often labelled flashbulb memory,[16] those with PTSD feel like they're constantly reliving their trauma. *Distracting* doesn't even begin to cover that. Paradoxically, PTSD often prevents you from actively recalling specific details of the event. It seems your brain, in a noble attempt at self-preservation, won't let you deliberately relive the known trauma. So, PTSD sometimes prevents you from *voluntarily* remembering the incident, which would be useful for processing it and coming to terms with it, but persistently makes you *involuntarily* remember it, when something around you randomly triggers memory. It's the worst of all worlds.

PTSD often results in hypervigilance, where you're constantly primed to recognise and respond to anything even vaguely threatening. It sounds like paranoia, and there undeniably are aspects of that, but it's a lot more persistent and powerful. It's basically having your threat detection system seriously amplified and maintaining dominance over most of your thoughts and reactions. This is the main process in most forms of anxiety, but it seems to be even stronger here, making it harder for individuals to push through or suppress it, even with much effort. This has knock-on effects, like trouble sleeping, irritability, poor concentration, and more.

Someone who regularly deals with PTSD and the many unpleasant effects of it is the actor, writer and comedian Bethany Black.

I don't really leave the house much. I do go to work and occasionally I'll go to the supermarket and if I do, then I have to have headphones in and sunglasses on and my phone next to me, so that I can focus on that to try and hide some of the rest of the world to reduce anxiety levels.

On a day-to-day basis, I can't really go anywhere and do anything. It becomes difficult as a result of that. The agoraphobia as a result of the PTSD has affected me in such a way, it's made me hypervigilant. The PTSD has gone in and put me in a situation where, when I'm out of the house, I'm certain that any person at any point could

*attack me. This is because my brain has figured out that
that's happened in the past and is likely to happen in the
future.*

*There is so little warning of it and there is so little ability
to figure out how it's going to be. The traditional sort of
cognitive behavioural therapy techniques of going out and
flooding* and repeatedly putting myself in that situation
don't help. On top of things like that and because of some
of the abuse that I've got – verbal abuse, emotional verbal
abuse – it's led me to become paranoid about certain
aspects of how I present myself and my voice, for example.*

Bethany's experiences are bad enough, but it doesn't end
there. Those dealing with PTSD can also experience issues
with their perception. Their senses become distorted, often
leading to things like hallucinations. Admittedly, there aren't
as many physiological symptoms needed to classify PTSD,
but the usual physical effects of severe anxiety are often there,
often during episodes when someone experiences the painful recall. All the symptoms described here should, according to the ICD criteria, occur within six months of the initial
incident, although delayed onset is not unheard of. The DSM
also states symptoms should be present for at least a month.[17]

All told, it could be argued that a brain with PTSD is one
that's essentially gone on the defensive, to the extreme. But

---

* The approach of exposing a patient to the source of their fears for prolonged periods, so they can adapt or become accustomed to them, having
been equipped with relaxation techniques and coping methods. A reasonably common approach, albeit an unpleasant one.

while such defensive measures by the threat detection system are meant to be helpful (in the evolutionary survival sense), anyone with PTSD will tell you that they really aren't. They're hugely disruptive and debilitating.

And that, in many ways, is at the root of all anxiety disorders – at least, according to available evidence. But before we get to that, there are few more anxiety disorders we should look at.

Social anxiety, phobias, and all the rest

Not every anxiety disorder is ever-present. Some are more discreet, more specific. Perhaps the most familiar anxiety disorder is *phobia*. Some estimates state that one in twenty people worldwide have a phobia of some sort.[18] You may well have one yourself. A specific phobia is when you have an intense anxiety reaction, with many physical symptoms like shortness of breath, shaking, nausea, and intense fear and panic, when presented with a specific stimulus or situation.

There are several classes of phobias. There are animal-type phobias: a fear of rats, dogs, snakes, spiders, etc. We've all heard about arachnophobia.* Then there are the natural environment phobias, such as a fear of naturally occurring things like water, aquaphobia, or heights, acrophobia. Situational phobias are a recognised form triggered by certain situations, most famously the fear of being in enclosed spaces, claustrophobia. There are also blood/injection/injury phobias, which are fears of those exact things.

---

* It was the title of a Hollywood film, after all.

Fear of clowns, or specific types of food, or, I don't know, lawnmowers? All these phobias come under the umbrella of 'simple' phobias, because it's relatively straightforward to see what causes them. Phobias that don't fit the main categories are labelled 'other' phobias.

Then there are *complex* phobias. Two in particular warrant mention. The first of these is social phobia, or social anxiety disorder, and is incredibly common.[19] We humans are an intensely social species, so much of our brain is geared towards making and maintaining relationships and gaining the approval of others. This is believed to stem from our tribal development in the wild, where our ability and desire to work together, to cooperate in large groups, made us the dominant species on Earth. But the fact that our survival hinged on being part of a group significantly affected how our brain evolved, as demonstrated by much of its internal workings.[20]

We have multiple networks and processes dedicated to facilitating social interactions and communication, like empathy and face recognition, and so on. The neurohormones oxytocin and vasopressin are primarily known for their properties of enhancing and sustaining emotional bonds between individuals. Parts of the brain heavily involved with processing social relationships, like the striatum, are closely linked to the reward pathway – the part of the brain that literally creates feelings of pleasure and well-being – which may explain why we take such comfort and enjoyment from interacting with others, in multiple contexts.

On the flip side, being dismissed or rejected by others, even if they're total strangers, has been shown to cause activity in those parts of the brain responsible for processing pain, hence we don't deal with rejection very well.[21] Indeed, much of our threat detection network and related processes are dedicated to recognising cues that are social in nature. Angry expressions, harsh tones, potential judgement and embarrassment, stuff like that. You can repeat that saying about sticks and stones all you like, but being insulted, or experiencing any other clear form of rejection, *does* hurt, at the most fundamental levels.

Because of all that, many people have genuine, deep-rooted fears and anxieties about doing something – anything – that could lead to embarrassment, rejection or unfavourable scrutiny. Public speaking is probably the most familiar example. But it can be speaking on the phone, paying for something at a checkout, eating in public. People can, and do, experience great anxiety about the mere thought of such things.*

When exposed to the trigger of their phobias, people invariably experience what looks like a panic attack. There are many of the same symptoms, like heart palpitations, trembling, sweating, nausea, sensations of choking, blushing, or fear of throwing up and/or soiling yourself. Interestingly, while disruptive and unpleasant, phobias usually only affect us when we're presented with the specific situation, or stimulation, that triggers them.

For instance, if you're phobic about public speaking, you will experience an attack if made to do public speaking, but

---

* Often with phobias, just thinking of the thing causes an anxious, fearful response. This is called anticipatory anxiety.

you'll be able to function fine in any other situation, so can live a normal life. But this isn't so easy for everyone. Say you're extremely phobic of snakes, but you live in London. How often would you encounter one of the legless reptiles? Pretty much never. Ergo, your life is largely unaffected.

But say you live in London and you're extremely phobic of birds, specifically pigeons?* London is teeming with them. Your life is going to be extremely stressful because every time you go outside, you're racked with fear and anxiety, because your feathery triggers are everywhere. And if your phobia is a social one, it's practically impossible to operate in the modern world without interacting with dozens of people on a regular basis, so you'll likely encounter your trigger more often. It becomes debilitating.

The second important complex phobia is agoraphobia. Many people believe agoraphobia is a fear of open spaces – even the name suggests this. It's derived from the Greek *agora*, meaning an open public place. Because of this, many think it is the opposite of claustrophobia. This, I stress, is wrong.

Agoraphobia is essentially a deep-rooted fear that a particular environment, or situation, is unsafe, and that you will be unable to get away from it.[22] This can apply to open spaces, to enclosed ones, to being part of a crowd, to being on public transport, and anything like that. Agoraphobia seems like a combination of intense social and intense situational phobias.

Individuals with agoraphobia also show pronounced avoidance behaviour, where they steer clear of anything,

* As many people are.

anywhere or anyone that could bring about an attack. But with agoraphobia, the range of potential triggers is very wide, so much so that afflicted individuals often end up sticking close to the only assured safe place, their home. In severe cases, some can only venture out in the company of someone they feel they can trust, and even then it's difficult. Others struggle to do even this much. Obviously, if someone can't face leaving their home, it's easily misread as them being afraid of open spaces, so the confusion persists.

Agoraphobia also has a lot of overlaps with panic disorder, given the very similar symptoms; the anxiety and apprehension, the preoccupation with experiencing an attack or episode. We heard from Bethany Black about dealing with agoraphobia on top of PTSD and other things. The DSM even goes so far as to distinguish between panic disorder *with* and *without* agoraphobia.

As I understand it, the main difference is that agoraphobia involves a powerful anxious reaction to feelings of helplessness and entrapment, which can come from almost anywhere, while panic disorder is more the experience of unexpected panic attacks, and persistent anxiety regarding the possibility of a panic attack. But in terms of how someone is affected by these things, they look objectively very similar, hence diagnosis must be quite particular about what is being dealt with.

And finally, there are other disorders worthy of an honourable mention in this anxiety chapter. Obsessive-compulsive disorder, the famous OCD, was previously deemed an anxiety disorder, due to the intense anxiety experienced by those with

OCD who are unable to satisfy or quell their compulsions, whatever they happen to be. However, the latest version of the DSM, the DSM-5, no longer lists OCD as an anxiety disorder.[23] It now has its own category of 'obsessive-compulsive and related' disorders; modern data show that the underlying brain mechanisms causing OCD are markedly different to those believed responsible for most anxiety disorders.

The anxiety experienced as part of OCD, while prominent, seems peripheral to the root cause of the issue, rather than the issue itself. At least, that's what the latest evidence suggests. Opinions on this differ, but it's enough for me to leave this issue aside for now.

Similarly, there's separation anxiety disorder, where severe anxiety occurs when separated from a specific person or place. You could argue that homesickness is a common, low-level manifestation of this. However, while reasonably common in adults, separation anxiety is mostly seen in very young children, which introduces a lot of considerations from child and developmental psychology and neuroscience, a whole other issue we don't really have space to cover right now.

As said earlier, the boundaries between what is and isn't deemed an anxiety disorder can fluctuate a lot, and this often comes back to the slippery criteria for what counts as a mental health problem. However, this discussion risks dragging us back to the philosophical and ideological debates surrounding mental health, none of which are going away any time soon. So, let's move on to something more physical. Specifically, what's happening in the brain when we experience clinical anxiety?

The neurological chemicals of anxiety

We've covered at length the sort of chemicals at work in the brain, both in general, and during depression. So, is there a particular chemical, or set of chemicals, underpinning the process of anxiety?

In many ways, no. Anxiety, like any other fabulously complex cognitive experience, can't really be reduced to, or explained purely in terms of, simple chemical actions. But, having said that, there *are* some chemicals worth flagging up, particularly because they're a big part of why anxiety can be so demanding and disruptive for your health, both mental and physical.

Most people label them stress hormones, those chemicals that are pumped round our body by a brain that is alert to threats and dangers thanks to the threat detection system, something we've discussed at length. The chemical cortisol[24] is often called *the* stress hormone, as it's released into our bloodstreams in significantly high levels at times of stress, and has numerous confirmed physiological effects on our tissues and organs. In fairness, it's actually one of a number of similar chemicals, called glucocorticoids, but it's the one that gets the most attention, so is sort of the spokesperson of the stress chemicals.[25]

Cortisol is yet another chemical signal that preps the body, and brain, to deal with adversity and imminent challenges. It affects our metabolism, causing us to better absorb and retain glucose and other energy sources. This makes sense; if you're about to deal with something challenging or dangerous, you don't want to risk running out of energy before you're done.

Cortisol also suppresses the immune system. This might sound counterproductive, because doesn't the immune system protect us, and keep us alive? Yes, but although a functioning immune system is vital, an immune response to injury or infection causes swelling and irritation and pain. You don't want that while you're tackling a threat, because it'll just slow you down. Hence cortisol, the stress chemical, suppresses the immune system response.

Cortisol has many other effects on our metabolism, but it also affects the brain, such as enhancing memory formation and focus. Because if you're tackling dangers, you don't want to be distracted, or forget what you learn about them, because this sort of thing might happen again.

There's also adrenaline, that well-known hormone that hits our bloodstream when we're scared, thrilled or otherwise worked up. Basically, when our threat detection system sounds the alarm, adrenaline starts flowing. It increases heart rate, muscle tension and strength, and a lot of studies have shown that it affects the brain by also enhancing memory and retrieval.[26]

Adrenaline also seems to increase negative emotions. It isn't just released in response to fear, adrenaline *keeps* us afraid/worried/anxious.[27] This is one way in which the anxiety response can be self-sustaining. Being anxious keeps us anxious, in other words. Remember that – it'll come up again soon.

The problem is that these chemicals, and those like them, are, in the evolutionary sense, meant to help us deal with threats. Which is great, and very helpful. But as discussed, for most of our history, threats were things that, for better or worse, went away. The point is, stress hormones, like cortisol and adrenaline etc., are only intended for short-term use.* Problems occur when short-term things hang around for a long time. It's like how leaving a car's engine running all night will deplete the fuel and hugely increase wear and tear, making problems and breakdowns more likely. Cortisol and adrenaline being a constant presence in our bodies means we experience their effects over the long term, meaning they stop being helpful, and start being harmful.

Cortisol's constant presence means our metabolism remains geared to conserving energy, largely by retaining calories, so we gain weight. Our immune systems remain suppressed, so healing wounds and infections takes longer than normal. Our muscles stay tense and blood pressure stays high, with all the accompanying health risks that brings. Our brains stay alert and focused, so we can't sleep, or relax, and remain constantly on edge.

Does that sound like anxiety to you? It should. With these stress chemicals lingering in our systems, we can start to see here how, and why, anxiety disorders have so many physical symptoms.

There are other chemicals gaining attention lately too, like neuropeptide Y, another stress chemical, this one released by the amygdala directly. It also has numerous roles in stress,[28]

---

* Insofar as anything set up by the unthinking process of evolution can be said to be *intended*.

but one noted property is that it's orexigenic.[29] In plain English, it increases appetite.*

The phenomenon of stress eating? This might explain that. Of course, with neuropeptide Y increasing our food intake and cortisol increasing our tendency to retain calories, it's no wonder stress and anxiety can lead to rapid weight gain.

And what controls release of cortisol? Our old friend, the HPA axis. And adrenaline? Would it be shocking to hear that the HPA axis – the hypothalamic-pituitary-*adrenal* axis – also controls the release of adrenaline? And what is it that causes the HPA axis to pump these stress chemicals into our bodies and brains? Usually, the amygdala. So, an overactive amygdala causes all these negative fearful emotions, which releases all these stress chemicals, profoundly affecting us on the physical and mental levels.

Having said all this, it could easily apply to a standard period of prolonged stress, a very common experience for many. It doesn't need to be an official anxiety disorder to be bad for us. So how, and why, does an anxiety *disorder* come about? How and why does the amygdala become so out of control?

The anxiety caused by a loss of control

If we accept that anxiety is largely down to an overactive amygdala and a prefrontal cortex that is somehow unable to rein it in . . . why would this happen? Well, these two regions

---

* Hence the term *anorexia*, to mean no appetite.

are precariously balanced at the best of times, constantly rubbing up against each other, and vying for dominance. This dominance is usually determined by what's happening at the time, the situation being dealt with. But in chronic anxiety issues, this balance is disrupted, and prefrontal cortex regions are seemingly hamstrung, letting the amygdala run amok, causing unhelpful and unnecessary stress and fear and panic and worry.

Why?

Well, obviously there can be many contributing factors. It's the brain, after all. However, there are a few intriguing possibilities raised by the available evidence.

You may think that the connections between the amygdala and prefrontal cortex, which the latter would logically need to send signals that control and regulate the former, are reduced, or limited in some way. We saw back in Chapter 2 that how effective a brain is at doing something is often determined by how well connected the regions involved in that particular process are. So, logically, if the prefrontal cortex connections to the amygdala are insufficient or reduced, that particular brain is going to have more difficulty in keeping the amygdala in check, so will be more prone to anxiety. Right?

It certainly could be for some people. Maybe some fluke of genes or an adverse developmental event means that their prefrontal cortex isn't as thoroughly linked to their amygdala as it should be. But there's much data showing that people with anxiety have *more* connections between the prefrontal cortex and amygdala, not fewer.[30]

It sounds weird, but remember, the brain isn't static; it's constantly changing, adapting. As such, if you make it do something constantly, the parts of the brain responsible for that task often increase and expand in response. Experienced London taxi drivers have bigger spatial navigation brain regions, concert pianists have larger brain areas dedicated to fine finger control. And people with anxiety have more connections between their prefrontal cortex and amygdala, presumably because they spend more time than anyone trying to shut their amygdala up!

Consciously, constantly and *actively* trying to suppress or limit the influence of the amygdala would logically mean there's a lot more activity between it and the prefrontal cortex. The neuroplasticity of the brain means that the connections that relay this activity would be deemed more important, so be expanded and enhanced. And thus, we end up with more of them.

You know the myth of Sisyphus? The deceitful king, cursed by the Greek gods to push a boulder up a hill, only to have it roll back down again, for all eternity? You'd assume that, after a few weeks of that, Sisyphus would be in very good physical shape. Constant, relentless exercise would mean his muscles would get much bigger. In modern terms, Sisyphus was probably pretty jacked. But . . . it didn't make a difference, did it? The boulder kept rolling down anyway. Similarly, the prefrontal cortex can have all the connections to the amygdala it likes. If the amygdala doesn't respond to signals telling it to stop causing stress and fear, they won't be any use.

So, something else seems to be going on. Something that makes the signals from the prefrontal cortex less effective.

Stop. GABA time! The crucial role of the inhibitor chemical

Earlier, we learned about glutamate, the neurotransmitter that accounts for most of the stimulation going on in the brain. With such a potent stimulating neurotransmitter so abundant in our brains, how does it ever stop doing anything? Well, there's another neurotransmitter, which has the opposite effect. Rather than *stimulating* neurons, causing them to generate more signals to make things happen, it *inhibits* them. It tells them to stop sending signals, and to ignore any neurotransmitter that argues otherwise. The neurotransmitter in question is officially named Gamma-Amino-Butyric-Acid, but everyone just calls it GABA. GABA is the major inhibitory neurotransmitter in the brain. It, and the neurons that use it, are the elements of the brain that tell other parts, 'No, stop doing that.'

This is an extremely important role. Think of the brain as a road network around a vast and busy city. GABA neurons are the red traffic lights. Yes, it's annoying to be stopped by one if you want to get somewhere, but imagine the carnage that would occur without them. GABA also seems to act differently to most neurotransmitters.[31] It effectively modifies the properties of a neuronal membrane, making it more porous, allowing more charged ions to cross back and forth, and so on. Unlike with most neurotransmitters, this doesn't change the voltage of the neuron membrane. But it makes it a lot harder to change the voltage, an essential step in neural signalling and activity.

Remember when I compared the signals in a neuron to ripples in the surface of a pond? Well, GABA essentially freezes the surface. You can still break through it, but you need much bigger, harder and heavier rocks. The little pebbles that are the normal excitatory neurotransmitters can't have the same effect they usually do. The neuron is effectively suppressed, shut down. That's how my old biology teacher explained it, anyway.

GABA has a prominent role throughout the brain, because most neurological processes need to be controlled. So, predictably, GABA has a key role in regulating emotional reactions, particularly stopping excessive ones. Unfortunately, we're only just beginning to understand the specific mechanisms of how GABA controls emotional experiences, and pretty much anything else. But there are still some interesting findings to consider. For instance, there are GABA neurons *within* the amygdala. A part of the amygdala, called the basolateral nucleus, is rich in GABA neurons, and extends these into other parts of the amygdala, to limit or suppress activity generated there.[32]

You could say this is the 'off' switch of the amygdala. And research reveals that many neural projections from the prefrontal cortex are connected to this region. This is how, presumably, those smarter parts of your brain usually exert control over the simpler, emotional activity generated by the amygdala.

There are also plenty of GABA neurons in the prefrontal cortex,[33] because a lot of activity goes on there, trying to make sense of everything that's going on in the brain, and much of this activity will be unhelpful or unnecessary. GABA neurons keep things under control there, too. This is particularly true in reactions to emotional stimuli. The prefrontal cortex works out what's a reasonable or unreasonable emotional response. The GABA system plays a key role in this process.

Here's an important point, though: GABA doesn't have a simple, yes/no, on/off effect. Its functions are many, diverse, and rather subtle. It's not like someone slamming on the brakes, bringing everything to a halt. Often, it refines and modifies key activity, so it's more like a sculptor, gradually and delicately chiselling away at a block of marble, to reveal an impressive, sophisticated, detailed statue. But imagine if the GABA system was hampered in some way. Imagine if all the red traffic lights suddenly went out. It's easy to see that this would quickly lead to things going wrong.

And many believe this is what happens in anxiety.[34] The crucial GABA neurons that keep everything running smoothly are somehow disrupted. So, those GABA neurons that keep the amygdala in check – the ones the prefrontal cortex relies on, to maintain control? They don't work so well. That's why the number of connections from the prefrontal cortex doesn't automatically mean reduced anxiety. It doesn't matter how many times you press the off switch if the switch itself doesn't work.

This GABA disruption, if it also affects the key GABA neurons found in the prefrontal cortex, could similarly skew the processing of emotional information, maybe amplifying how potent emotions are, particularly fearful and anxious ones, in the more conscious parts of the brain. Indeed, if the GABA system is hampered throughout the whole brain, you'd expect to see more activity overall. The teacher's left the room, and the unruly kids are running wild.

Anxiety is, at the most basic level, an excess of activity in key regions of the brain. For instance, the drug ketamine, discussed previously in the context of how it powerfully stimulates the glutamate system, can cause sensory disruption with even moderate doses.[35] These sensory problems are very similar to those experienced by people with PTSD.

When a drug that strongly increases brain activity has the same consequences as a serious anxiety disorder, it's hard not to argue that there's some similar mechanism at work in both. And, perhaps predictably, the disruption of the glutamate system can result in increased activity of the HPA axis, our old friend who causes many of the physical and mental consequences of prolonged stress. But, once again, every answer just leads to further questions. If it is the disruption of the GABA system that results in all the disruptive amygdala activity that leads to all the problems of anxiety, why is the GABA system disrupted in the first place?

One possibility is that it's down to neurosteroids.

The steroids of the brain and their role in anxiety

A very complex group of chemicals, neurosteroids have many diverse roles, as well as invariably long and complex names that would make this book even more confusing if I included them here. Neurosteroids, as the name suggests,

219

are produced throughout the brain, usually by glia, those support cells attached to neurons that maintain and protect them.*

Essentially, neurosteroids are an integral part of the support cells' role in keeping neurons and their specific properties working. But it's believed that they often also induce the changes that allow neurons to adapt and modify. Principally, neurosteroids play a key role in plasticity.[36] It would require a whole other book to explore in detail the work of neurosteroids in the brain, but in this context, they seem to play a key role in maintaining GABA neurons and their functioning.[37] Via complex interactions with the specific receptors, certain neurosteroids modulate, or refine, the actions of GABA, according to what's needed.

And here's the thing; evidence suggests that neurosteroids enhance and reinforce the GABA system during *acute* stress, meaning stress that's immediate and substantial. But neurosteroids seem to decline, and stop maintaining the GABA neurons, in response to chronic, *prolonged* stress.[38]

Why? Well, maybe it's another consequence of how the stress system was never meant to operate long term. Perhaps support cells simply run out of neurosteroids, being unable to maintain a supply in the face of constant demand. While the powerful human intellect means we *can* stay worried and anxious over long periods, at the basic cellular level this is unsustainable. So, neurosteroids decline, the inhibitory GABA

---

* Back in Chapter 2 I said I wasn't going to talk about them again, but it turns out I was wrong. I hope you'll forgive me this mistake.

system suffers, excess brain activity caused by fear and worry isn't curbed, worry and stress and anxiety become prolonged and unshakable, and there we have anxiety disorder.

The frustrating diversity of the anxious brain

I'll emphasise this important point again: there is no one easy explanation for any mental health problem, particularly one as complex and versatile as anxiety. But even if we could pin it all on one specific underlying mechanism, such as the neuro-steroids, GABA, amygdala overactivity model I just outlined, that doesn't mean we can reliably predict and understand *all* anxiety disorders. There's just too much going on in the brain. For instance, why do some people succumb to anxiety, while others don't? There seem to be genetic factors at work, so a family history is a part of it. Some people seemingly have a susceptibility to anxiety in their DNA.[39]

But also, those unhelpful chemical changes that occur in response to stress? They can happen at early ages too. So, if you have a particularly stressful childhood or upbringing, this will impact on how your brain develops, so the negative changes brought by stress, such as a more active, less controllable amygdala, become more lasting and permanent, like a house built on slightly unstable foundations, potentially leaving you more prone to stress issues and subsequent anxiety.[40] Such factors are believed to play a role in the development of things like borderline personality disorder, too. The many, many layers of complexity involved in the development and formation of the brain mean it's

221

impossible to predict with any accuracy how things will pan out.

But the ever-expanding body of anxiety research is constantly finding signs that the brain reacts to constant stress and activity in different ways, and this may underpin the many different expressions of anxiety disorders. For example, recent evidence suggests that brains with panic disorder have an HPA axis that's particularly sensitive to *novel* situations that imply danger and threat.[41]

Our brains are very keen on novelty. How unfamiliar, how new, a thing is can readily enhance how quickly and how strongly we react to it. Whatever that reaction may be. It can be a good thing, like finding a tenner in the pocket of some old trousers. This often feels more rewarding than having your monthly pay go into your bank account. The pay is a greater amount, but you weren't *expecting* the trouser money. It's not familiar. Novel. Therefore, more rewarding.

But it can be bad too. Think of jump-scares, that classic horror tactic where something *unexpected* occurs in an already tense situation. This is invariably much more frightening. The unexpected, the novel, enhances the fear response too. And it seems that the stress response in the brain of someone with panic disorder is particularly sensitive to novelty. This could explain why panic attacks are so unpredictable. If they're triggered by novel, unfamiliar things, *of course* you wouldn't be able to anticipate what sets them off. And we saw earlier that a lot of the activity of the amygdala and threat detection system happens too quickly for the complex regions like the prefrontal cortex to get involved with. Perhaps that's happening here?

Maybe that's why it's hard to pin down what actually set it all off. And because you don't anticipate it, you can't prepare yourself for it. So, when something novel does happen, your instinctive systems kick in and go from zero to sixty right away.

Basically, panic disorder may arise when you're set off by something new, something unfamiliar, and your fight-or-flight systems scramble to catch up, turning everything up to maximum, just to be safe. Hence, panic attacks. It's one possible explanation.

Other studies suggest that an overactive amygdala can have excessive influence on regions and processes responsible for interpreting social cues and actions, like the superior temporal gyrus, thalamus, and, as ever, the prefrontal cortex.[42] These regions are regularly assessing the behaviour of those around you and interpreting what it means. But if the amygdala is having too much input, they interpret social situations with an excessively fearful, paranoid slant. If all social situations seemed ominous and worrisome to you, social anxiety would be a logical outcome.

Other data imply that other areas, like the striatum and anterior cingulate cortex, are involved in recognising negative social cues, like angry expressions or stand-offish body language. These also seem to be more active in people with social anxiety disorder, meaning we become hyper-aware of unpleasant social interactions, even if they're only *possible* ones. Could this be down to the suppressed GABA system, meaning multiple parts of the brain are more active than they should be? Possibly. Either way, it makes us more socially anxious. And this can have knock-on effects.

Earlier, I said we have dedicated neurohormones, oxytocin and vasopressin, that enhance our emotional bonds with other people. Well, some studies show that these chemicals suppress activity in the amygdala. This would explain why we feel safer, more relaxed, when surrounded by those we like, or love, or trust. We even covered how people with agoraphobia can often only venture out if accompanied by someone they trust implicitly, and perhaps this explains that, too.

Of course, if you have serious social anxiety, you practise avoidance behaviours. You steer clear of others, forgo relationships and interactions, so the amygdala isn't suppressed by such actions and thus remains at full, excessive, strength.

There are other things that can prolong anxiety, or make it self-sustaining. The long-suffering prefrontal cortex: we've seen how it's largely responsible for making sense of everything that's going on in the brain, for giving us a coherent perception, a narrative of sorts.[43] Well, one possibility is that, during anxiety, it's constantly trying to make sense of all the anomalous, excessive activity going on in the brain; as if it notes the elevated amygdala activity and says, 'That must mean there's danger, but I can't spot it, so just stay alert.' This would explain the general anxiety in generalised anxiety disorder; it's the smarter parts of the brain trying to impose a logical response on what it's experiencing, but can't pin it on anything specific. Maybe that's how adrenaline increases fear and anxiety? The prefrontal cortex notes the elevated adrenaline levels, and thinks 'I must be worried about something, otherwise this wouldn't be there,' and we experience things accordingly.

There are other ways this can play out. When it comes to tackling challenges or threats, there are two separate motivation systems in the brain: *approach*, which compels us to deal with the problem, tackle it head-on; and *avoid,* which makes us want to steer clear of it. Fight or flight, respectively. What if the increased activity of anxiety affects one more than the other, throwing the balance off?

That would explain a lot. If the avoid system is overstimulated, we'd feel compelled to steer clear of anything threatening. But maybe *everything* feels threatening? Because anxiety often does that. This would explain a lot of avoidant behaviour, even agoraphobia.

Alternatively, the approach system could be more stimulated. A lot of people with anxiety report a desperate need to keep busy, to stay on top of things, to take on more. They're restless, on edge, all the time, frantically trying to retain control of their lives. If the part of your brain that compels you to deal with things is overly active, but for no obvious reason, this behaviour could be the result.

Also, an active threat detection system, plus an energised approach system in the brain, is usually something that results in, or is caused by, anger. And many people with anxiety report persistent irritability and anger.[44] Maybe this explains that? Maybe the confused prefrontal cortex notes the energised threat detection and approach systems and thinks, 'I guess I must be angry about something'.

Again, this is mostly speculation, based on snippets of the vast ocean of available data. The brain is amazingly complex, flexible and chaotic, and the diversity of anxiety disorders reflects that as well as anything. But that isn't to say anxiety is completely beyond our understanding. Because it isn't. The fact is, there are numerous effective treatments available, and that further helps our understanding of anxiety, as well as other mental health problems.

The depression and anxiety overlap

There are numerous therapeutic interventions available for those with anxiety disorders, depending on what they are and how they manifest. But, much like with antidepressants and other depression treatments, there's no guarantee that they'll definitely work. Each brain remains different, and responds to things in very specific, unpredictable ways. However, speaking of depression, when it comes to medication, the most common, and usually reliable, treatment for anxiety is . . . antidepressants. SSRIs, specifically.[45]

How come? Well, you've likely noticed* that much of what's been discussed in this chapter on anxiety was already mentioned in the previous chapter on depression. But the two disorders do indeed have a lot of features in common. Perhaps they even stem from a similar issue in the brain?

We explored the idea that depression is due to a loss of neuroplasticity, when the neurons in key areas are essentially exhausted. Prolonged, excessive activity, caused by the stress system, leaves our brains unable to alter or improve mood. But isn't a period of prolonged, excessive, stress-induced

* Because I've pointed it out repeatedly.

activity pretty much exactly what anxiety is? Could it be that anxiety is the thing that causes a brain to become depressed? Indeed, most people who experience both anxiety and depression report that anxiety occurs first. And in the developing, adolescent brain, anxiety is more common in the earlier years, and depression in the later teens.

Undoubtedly, there are stark differences between depression and anxiety. Anxiety is essentially the constant feeling that something awful *could* happen, while depression is more feeling that something awful *has* happened/*is* happening. Someone with depression invariably lacks energy or motivation, while someone with anxiety often has too much, in a nervous, unhelpful way. But this is still consistent with the idea that anxiety is the period of high activity that damages the plasticity of neurons, leading to depression.

Not every person with depression experiences anxiety first, of course. But maybe they're more susceptible to stress and the like, so it takes less harmful activity to hamper their mood-regulating processes? So, maybe they experience depression without displaying full-blown anxiety. Remember, diagnosis can be a limited, variable process at the best of times, and the anxiety symptoms need to be present for six months before being officially confirmed. There's plenty of wiggle room.

Even in the underlying circuitry of the brain, there's overlap. Some studies show that those with both depression and anxiety, a very common expression of poor mental health, have a particularly sensitive, overactive HPA axis,[46] so are particularly reactive to stressful things. Hence, the same medication often works for both anxiety and depression.

227

There's no definitive answer as to *why* SSRIs are effective for both disorders. It could be that the way SSRIs enhance the ability to control and regulate mood has a similar role in limiting anxiety. Perhaps they give the prefrontal cortex more power over the amygdala, allowing it to wrest back control over your inner workings?

Other studies suggest that our instinctive tendency to avoid or recoil from anything deemed harmful and threatening is disrupted in both anxiety and depression, so both disorders make it harder to avoid encountering and consciously thinking about such things. This leads to substantial stress, and we know by now what that does to us. This instinctive recoil process is seemingly supported by the serotonin system, so boosting serotonin may give us back our tendency to avoid stressful things without having to think about them. And thinking about all the bad things that could, or do happen, is another thing that depression and anxiety have in common.

Another possibility is that SSRIs increase output of neurosteroids.[47] This takes a while, hence both anxiety and depression symptoms are only alleviated weeks after taking SSRIs, not right away. But when it does happen, the neurosteroids get the GABA systems working again, so all the unpleasant, harmful, stressful processes running rampant in the brain in both depression and anxiety can be knocked back, at last.

Maybe it's all these things? Or something else entirely? Research is, as ever, ongoing. But all this we've just discussed, and more besides, reveals that there's a growing

228

body of evidence that suggests seemingly different mental disorders, like depression and anxiety, have common roots.

The many ways of tackling anxiety

This isn't to say there aren't drugs for tackling anxiety specifically. The anxiolytic drugs, to give them their official title, are well known. And they usually work. Actually, they tend to work *too well*. The most common anxiolytics used today are the benzodiazepines, a diverse range of drugs of which the most famous is probably diazepam, aka Valium. They're known to be effective against pretty much every type of anxiety disorder. These drugs produce a powerful, and immediate, sedative effect. They're tranquillisers: they calm you down, relax you, stop you from worrying. They cancel out anxiety, basically. And they do this by increasing the effects of GABA, the neurotransmitter system that suppresses or stops things happening in the brain.[48] These drugs give it a powerful boost, so it can finally shut down all the excess activity of anxiety. They also work for sleep disorders, for similar reasons.

But these drugs affect *all* of the brain, not just the bits you want dealt with. Other parts that get suppressed include your higher reasoning abilities – hence things like Valium tend to leave you very relaxed, almost spaced out, as thinking straight becomes a lot harder. And because they shut down a lot of the stress and anxiety systems, that often makes them very enjoyable. Simultaneously, they're so potent, the effect they have on the brain is so strong, that the brain responds in kind, rapidly changing and adapting in ways that make benzodiazepines very addictive.[49] Therefore, they're used sparingly, and cautiously.

Perhaps this is inevitable when it comes to drugs that treat anxiety symptoms directly. You're not trying to spark something that isn't there, like in depression. No, you're trying to suppress something that *is* there. This can be a much more risky, hazardous task, like rewiring a plug while the current's still running. There are other drugs that help anxiety, via different mechanisms. Opiates are sometimes used, what with the powerful painkiller effects they have being linked to pleasure and relaxation, something anxiety doesn't feature much of. Ditto cannabis.

However, anxiety treatment isn't limited to drugs. In low-level cases, some basic lifestyle changes can help. I emphasise the word *help*, not *cure* or *fix*, because if the problem exists deep within your brain then surface-level adjustments likely won't reach that far. But still, things like cutting down on caffeine, stopping smoking, better sleep, more exercise, etc., can help lower the excessive activity that is the main engine of anxiety.

Girl on the Net found such approaches worked for her:

One of the biggest things I learnt in counselling this year is just do less. I essentially have this habit of filling up my entire diary hour by hour, every single day, trying to make sure that every single thing I do in my life is productive in some way, working towards a goal. Like maintaining this friendship, or getting this bit of work done, doing this, that or the other, to the point where I'm cramming so much into all of my time, I never have any time to just relax and clear my mind.

Over the last year, the things that have made the biggest difference have been firstly that I took up a hobby that doesn't involve sitting behind a screen, and that I just enjoy doing for the sake of it. So, I'm doing quite a lot of woodwork at the moment, which is very nice. I made a cracking table! The other thing is that my counsellor this year – who was absolutely brilliant – as soon as I arrived at her place, she put in place a plan for me which was basically making sure I did three things every day that were just for pleasure. She also banned me from doing pretty much any of my work that wasn't necessary to pay my mortgage and my bills, just for a short period of time while I got into the habit of relaxing.

I've gone from working about fifty to sixty hours a week, down to about thirty hours. A lot of that is just about managing what I do. It took me a really long time to get to grips with that, and also to accept that it was okay, because ever since I was quite young I've always had this clock ticking in my head, going, 'You have to do more; you have to work harder.' And actually, sometimes I do have to relax.

Of course, this is assuming your anxiety isn't so bad that you are unable to do these things. Which often isn't the case. Having a therapist who can and will put a plan in place for you to impose structure on your brain can be a big help, but, as ever, there's no guarantee that it'll take, or prove effective.

Cognitive therapies – one-on-one counselling sessions – are known to be particularly effective for anxiety. Regular therapy sessions with trained experts can be helpful in getting you to process your stresses and worries in different, less anxiety-prompting ways. A lot of the psychological approaches to anxiety disorders could be said to be variations on the concept of teaching the afflicted brain to think about, or process, the triggers of anxiety, in new, alternative ways. Specifically, ways that don't trigger a stress or fear response. Despite how many clichés insist otherwise, the reason phobias can't be cured by facing your fears is that, when doing so, the brain learns the wrong lesson.

Someone with a serious arachnophobia knows that the tiny spider on the other side of the room doesn't really pose any threat. But their threat detection system isn't listening to the rational parts of the brain; it sees a spider, it goes into high alert, causing all the serious panic-attack-style symptoms. And the simpler, more fundamental parts of the brain learn by making connections. So, rather than 'I encountered a spider and nothing happened,' the phobic brain thinks 'I encountered a spider and my body and brain went absolutely haywire, therefore spiders *are* dangerous, and my fear is justified.'

The trick for this and many other relevant psychotherapies is to get the anxious brain to approach and process the usual triggers in ways that sidestep the threat detection system, thus avoiding the damaging fear and stress it causes. PTSD is particularly well researched here, given how it's one of the more serious anxiety disorders, with a clear, obvious cause. Prolonged exposure therapy is said to be the gold standard for PTSD,[50] where the individual is guided by the therapist to think about, or write about, or discuss the things that traumatised them, in safe and guided ways. As the therapy progresses, they may interact with known triggers of episodes, but again, in safe, manageable contexts. Hopefully, the brain learns to deal with the traumatic triggers, without being traumatised.

A similar treatment, known as systematic desensitisation,[51] or graduated exposure therapy, addresses severe phobias. It involves exposing someone to the source of their phobias, but in small, manageable increments that don't trigger a fear response. Take the person with severe arachnophobia that we just mentioned. For them, over a series of sessions, you'd maybe start by showing them a drawing of a small spider.

Then a photo of a small spider.

Then a video of a small spider.

Then a picture of a big spider.

Then a video of a big spider.

Then put them next to a fake small spider.

Then a big fake spider.

Then put them in a room with a small spider in a glass case.

And so on, and so on, until you reach the point where they're juggling tarantulas with a smile on their face.*

The process at work here is the same as that uncovered by Pavlov's famous dogs: classical conditioning. The anxious

---

* This is a joke. Nobody ever literally has to do this.

brain has learned that something equals a threat, so triggers a fear response whenever it encounters that something. It's the therapist's job to convince, or train, or condition the brain to recognise that the something equals no threat, so needn't be reacted to at all.

Obviously, that's a lot harder to achieve than this simple description suggests. Effective approaches vary from person to person, as in many cases the fear association is complex and deep, and each patient has such different thinking and cognition. And a lot of the time, the anxiety isn't linked to any one particular thing, i.e. generalised anxiety disorder. It's very hard to sever a connection when you can't even find it in the first place.

Consequently, a number of more modern therapies involve essentially distracting the anxious brain, or disrupting the emotional fear response, in other ways. Eye movement desensitisation and reprocessing, EMDR, is an increasingly popular, though still controversial, therapy, where patients are coached to make certain eye movements, a wholly unrelated neurological process that, in theory, takes resources and focus away from the disruptive aspects of processing traumatic emotions.[52] Some claim it works very well, others dispute the validity of the evidence, and the exact mechanism as to how this works, if indeed there is one, remains unclear.

Another, perhaps more straightforward, approach is biofeedback, or neurofeedback. It's where a patient is hooked up to a monitor that displays their body's vitals and outputs, such as heart rate, blood pressure and so on, or to an electroencephalograph (EEG), a machine that displays their relevant brainwaves. These levels and brainwaves noticeably change when someone is feeling anxious, or feels an attack coming on. But showing these changing levels, this *feedback*, directly to the patient gives the anxiety a more tangible, more visible aspect. So, rather than trying to suppress the emotional response, something we know is difficult, they can try to suppress the change in their biological responses or brainwaves.

Basically, they can see that their heart rate has gone up, so they can focus on trying to consciously lower it. Ditto specific brainwaves. To an extent, it removes the subjective feelings of anxiety and stress from the process, so a person can, hopefully, learn to counteract the effects of anxiety by alternative means, without relying on the impaired or disrupted system and networks where the emotions are dealt with directly.

It could be said that there is a common approach to EMDR, neurofeedback and just about anything that helps take away feelings of anxiety, from meditation to exercise to hobbies: they seem to shift the focus in the brain away from the emotional, anxiety-inducing reactions and towards more neutral, harmless ones. Also, the human brain seems to thrive on a sense of control; feeling in control is known to reduce levels of stress, so it could be that just doing something, anything, helps with this.

People with anxiety may well find their own unique ways to assert control. For example, here's Lowri Williams's approach:

In terms of my anxiety, to keep that under control, I do tactile things. I'll go and hold something hot, or cold, or I have paperclips in a little part of my desk at work – I'll pick them up and I'll count them. It just helps me ground, and control, and find something else, and then I'll move on.

At night when it's stopping me sleeping, I play an alphabet game. I'll pick a subject – boys' names, films, songs – and I'll go through the alphabet and try to think of a song or anything beginning with each letter. I usually find myself drifting off around about P or Q.

Of course, not every method of gaining a sense of control is automatically a good one, as Rachel England explains . . .

While I did it often in my teens, there have been maybe in the last ten years, a handful of times where I have actually self-harmed again. I wish that that wasn't the case, but for me I find it is one of the only ways that I can pull myself out of the mental state that I am in at the time. And just to be clear, I'm not suicidal. Self-harm isn't about suicide ideation; it's about control.

For me, because of my panic disorder, it's a way that makes my brain go, 'Oh my God, there's an injury on your body. Let's focus on that now.' It pulls me out of the panic spiral that I'd be in otherwise.

The problem here is that self-harming isn't a helpful solution by any means; it can easily make matters far worse. But the point is, when it comes to anxiety, a lot of the time we *don't*

236

have control over it, or our own fear-inducing emotions. So, we try to regain it, sometimes via radical, dangerous means. But there's no guarantee that we can succeed on our own.

That's one of the big reasons why anxiety is as much of a problem as it is.

The overall view of anxiety

So, what have we learned about anxiety?

It's very common and happens to literally everyone. But in some people, it happens too much, in ways that can't be stopped or curtailed without external help. And this causes problems. It seems to stem from an excess of activity, specifically in the amygdala, the source of feelings of fear and threat, and the rest of the brain is affected accordingly. Anxiety is another disorder that looks to be initially triggered by a stress response taken to excess, in this case the disruption of the GABA system, which quiets the brain down and keeps it under control. This may be the result of prolonged stress causing depletion and disruption to the release of neurosteroids, which usually keep the GABA system in shape.

It has a lot in common with depression, despite some notable differences. It may even be the cause of depression, in some cases. Depression and anxiety have a lot of fundamental processes that they share, in any case. Anxiety can, and does, manifest in a wide variety of ways, depending on how it begins, which parts of the brain are affected, and how the overall system processes and reacts to the underlying problem. Anxiety can be very specific, restricted to a single phobic trigger like spiders or enclosed spaces, or constant and widespread, as with panic disorder, generalised anxiety disorder and PTSD. The latter are undeniably more debilitating, and require more care and attention, but there's no *good* anxiety disorder, of course. That would make no sense.

There are a number of ways and means of addressing anxiety, but how effective they are depends on the specific nature of the anxiety, because each brain is different. That can't be stressed enough. There are drugs that deal with the symptoms, but they're fairly powerful and potentially disruptive in their own right, so should be used very carefully indeed.

There's actually a great deal more that could be said. Even this lengthy chapter has barely scratched the surface of all that's known, or suspected, about anxiety disorders. But at least we can take some comfort from the fact that our understanding of them is constantly expanding, so treatment and solutions are ever more likely. And perhaps there are some clues as to the fundamental roots of mental health problems in general.

It's far from certain, but there's mounting evidence to suggest that both anxiety and depression are the end result of an excessive and prolonged stress response, something that, in a cruel irony, probably wouldn't be an issue if we didn't have these big powerful brains that always find something to be anxious about.

Maybe the real answer to dealing with global depression and anxiety rates is simply to make the world a place that has fewer things to worry about? However, looking around at things in 2020, that doesn't seem likely any time soon.

5: Addiction

In Chapter 3, we looked at mood disorders, with an obvious and necessary emphasis on depression. In Chapter 4, it was anxiety disorders, and the many, many forms they can take. We've explored these conditions in extensive – some might say punishing – depth. But, I'd argue, for good reason. Because if you added up all the people in the world with depression and/or anxiety, you'd have over half a billion people. That's about seven per cent of the actual human species.

However, this leads back to a point I made back in the introduction: if these problems are so widespread, so commonplace, why is there still so much stigma attached to them? As highlighted back in that chapter, five times more people worldwide are affected by anxiety and depression than have red hair. Sure, having red hair can be the subject of mild mockery,* but overall, when compared to a more coppery hair colour, it's still the substantially more common mental health issues that attract suspicion, condemnation, judgement, interference, abuse, dismissal, and more. While mental health awareness campaigns are constantly chipping away at this, the stigma around mental health problems remains substantial. This is a problem, because such stigma makes things worse than they already are.

---

* Usually from people with a sense of humour about as sophisticated as that of a damp brick.

Stigma doesn't just appear when someone experiences a mental health episode, taking them by surprise. No, it's a constant, and widespread, part of everyday life. Every clueless attention-seeking pundit mocking those with depression, every scornful tabloid mention of 'happy pills', every familial conversation that downplays or dismisses someone's mental health concerns, every public condemnation of a suicide victim as selfish, every expression of concern or disbelief that someone is *still* taking medication, what with all the Big Pharma lies. All these things, and more, are examples of stigma, adding more shame and judgement to the very notion of poor mental health, and attempts to deal with it. And they all add up.

Such views and ever-present judgements shape how we interpret the world, influencing our understanding and expectations, leaving many with the impression that mental health problems are much more shameful than they are, that those experiencing them are inferior beings, flawed on some fundamental level. This affects everyone, to some extent. Families and friends, who would ideally form a necessary support network for someone dealing with poor mental health, may be less able (or less *willing*) to do so, thanks to stigma. The chronic underfunding of mental health services, and many reports of abuse and mistreatment of patients by those who work in them, shows that people can stigmatise mental health problems even when it's their literal job to take them seriously. All of this negatively affects those with poor mental health.

But also, consider this: if you've been led to believe that a mental health problem is a sign of weakness, or not really a big deal, or that it leads to scorn and rejection, how do you react if you end up with one? When your own mental health declines to the point where you can no longer function? You might deny it, even to yourself, desperately hoping that it goes away or fixes itself. But even if you *can* accept that you have a problem, you may still desperately try to hide it from others, for fear of their reaction.

In either case, denying a mental health problem (knowingly or unknowingly) thanks to stigma results in a far more demanding life, and therefore a significantly more stressful life. And we've seen, repeatedly, how bad prolonged stress is for your mental health. So, denying a mental health problem is far more likely to make it worse.

Following on from this, if someone is reluctant/unable to even admit that their mental health is not good, they're logically not going to seek help for it. So, thanks to stigma, countless mental health problems are made much worse, and ignored or left untreated, for far longer than is ideal.

However, those with mental health problems aren't helpless, passive victims. They, like everyone else, will do whatever they can to feel better. Because we all self-medicate. If you take paracetamol for a headache, or over-the-counter remedies for a cold, or even try mint tea for an upset stomach, you're self-medicating. You're addressing your own health issues *without* medical supervision.

For minor or fleeting problems, this is usually fine. But when it's a serious and chronic mental health problem, it often backfires. Tackling a mental health problem is a prolonged, complex process, involving much trial and error by many trained experts. It isn't really something that can be figured out by a single untrained individual, *while they're experiencing a mental health problem*. That can be like teaching yourself to fly a plane while you're in one, alone, as it's hurtling towards the ground. And yes, there's the piloting analogy again. But it remains relevant, so I keep using it.

Basically, self-medicating for mental health problems is typically limited to short-term relief. However, our world contains a lot of options for short-term relief. There are activities, experiences, even devices, that can make you feel good, or better, in short bursts. But usually, people opt for certain *substances*. Things like alcohol, caffeine and nicotine are available wherever you look. And if you're willing, or desperate enough, to ignore the law, there are numerous illegal drugs, which offer brief respite from whatever's going on in your head.

But I stress the phrase *short-term relief* because that's usually all you can hope for. If you start to rely on things like drink and drugs to make you feel better, you get a whole new set of problems, which, again, makes matters worse.

Therefore, in this penultimate chapter, we're going to look at addiction. Or substance misuse, or drug dependence, or however else it's defined. (That's actually an important aspect of it, which we'll get to in due time.)

Why addiction specifically? Well, firstly, some statistics argue that as many as thirty per cent of all people diagnosed with a mental health problem, regardless of what it is, also end up abusing alcohol or drugs. This figure rises as high as fifty per cent in those with severe mental health issues.[1] Granted, abusing alcohol and drugs isn't technically the same as being addicted, but it's an alarmingly short hop between them. Basically, if any and all mental health problems can increase the odds of addiction, it's undoubtedly very relevant.

As someone unfortunate enough to have ended up with a whole suite of mental health issues, Bethany Black can certainly vouch for the increased risk of addiction.

When I first got diagnosed with depression, I think I was twenty. I was at university and I'd kind of figured out that I had depression, only I thought I was faking it. I thought I was faking it for attention.

I had been self-harming since I was thirteen. I had been in a long-term-relationship that had broken up quite badly. I was twenty and we'd been together for about four years, so it was a big chunk of our very formative years, and it had fallen apart quite spectacularly.

There was no way of escaping it on any level at any time. I was drinking lots to try and cope and things just reached a point where I dissociated. Previously, whenever anything went wrong, my brain's impulse would be to drink, take some drugs. Deal with it that way.

It was the fake confidence from drugs and alcohol that would allow me not to have to panic, not to have to worry so much. Getting clean and sober has been a massive positive effect on my life. Dealing with the underlying causes of that has been great. However, some of the symptoms – some of the reasons why I did it – are a lot more complex to try to unpack and to get rid of.

Another more fundamental reason for focusing on addiction is that the disorders we've covered so far seem to stem from the human brain experiencing too much stress, something it doesn't like, for too long. Addiction shows us that the opposite isn't great either; experiencing something the brain *does* like, that it finds pleasurable, too frequently and for too long, also causes serious problems. It's not all about the stress response, although that does play a role in the consequences of addiction, as we'll see.

And finally, if there's one thing that shows how stigma directly affects mental health, it's addiction. There are still many people who refuse to accept that it is a mental health condition at all, and the stigma has profound and direct impacts on how it's dealt with and discussed. Given that this whole book is intended to increase understanding and reduce the stigma of mental health, addiction is a very useful thing to focus on.

So, with that in mind, let's look at how addiction works in the brain, how it's understood, and why it causes the problems it does, both internally and societally. Suffice to say, it's so much more than just a lack of willpower.

What *is* addiction?

The terms addiction and addicted are very common these days.

There's barely a day without some histrionic article declaring how children and young people are addicted to their smartphones, or social media, or devices in general.

244

High-profile, powerful men being outed for using their position to physically force themselves on women without their consent is a depressingly common occurrence, but in many cases the perpetrator's excuse is that they're addicted to sex.

When I was growing up, my own mother said I was addicted to the arcade machine we had in the pub we lived in. Because a young boy in a remote rural village in the mid-1980s constantly wanting to play the only video game within fifteen miles was clearly experiencing a pathological disorder. Basically, the term addiction is used a lot. But it *shouldn't* be. Because much of what people describe as addiction . . . isn't.

This overuse of the term can be disrespectful, even harmful, because addiction is a serious thing, not to be taken lightly. It can cause severe problems for an individual's health (mental and physical), their relationships, their prospects, their life in general, and often the lives of those around them. Therefore, using it to describe someone spending too much time on social media, according to some unspecified personal preference, is devaluing the term somewhat. It undermines and belittles anyone with a genuine addiction. And there we have that stigma again.

So, what *does* count as addiction? Genuine addiction is most common, by some margin, in the context of people who use and abuse psychoactive substances, to a chronic, disruptive and damaging degree. Drugs, basically.

A psychoactive substance, also known as a psychotropic substance, is one that, when introduced into one's body, affects the brain and nervous system, causing changes in mental processes. They make us think differently, feel differently, experience different emotions or perceptions. There's a very wide range of them.

However, not every psychoactive substance is automatically deemed a dangerous drug. Caffeine is a psychoactive drug. It makes us more awake, more focused, than we were before ingesting it. But it's not illegal, nor carefully regulated by medical professionals. No, it's widely available. High streets have a Starbucks or similar coffee chain on every corner. And countless people are open and proud of their love of, and dependence on, coffee. This doesn't mean it's not a psychoactive substance, it's just an *acceptable* one.

Of course, something being socially acceptable doesn't mean it's harmless. Caffeine dependence and withdrawal are things, don't doubt it.[2] Similarly, a colleague who worked in the addiction clinic at the nearby hospital informed me it could justifiably be renamed the alcoholism clinic, maybe 'Alcohol, and Friends', because the vast majority of patients were dealing with alcoholism.

Does this mean alcohol is the 'worst' drug? The most addictive? Probably not, no. But it's *the easiest to get*. And in much of modern culture, drinking alcohol isn't just accepted, it's encouraged. Consider all the different ways in which consuming alcohol is the expected norm. Weddings, birthdays, Christmas, work parties, dates, social gatherings; in situations like these, it's saying you *don't* want alcohol that's more likely to be met with suspicion and concern (in the UK, at least). The point is, psychoactive substances don't automatically lead to addiction. Often, they're just par for the course, a facet of everyday life.

So, where is the line crossed? How do you know when someone is addicted? What's the difference between casual or recreational use and a genuine problem?

Let's look at the criteria.

The latest edition of the DSM, the DSM-5, lists the following as necessary for a diagnosis in the substance-related and addictive disorders category. Essentially, do any of the following apply to you? Then you may have an addiction.

1. Taking more of a substance, or for longer periods, than initially planned, or hoped.

2. Intending or attempting to cut down or reduce use of a substance, but being unable to do so.

3. Dedicating a disproportionate amount of time to substance use, whether by obtaining, consuming, or recovering from it. For example, spending most of your waking hours in the pub, and always enduring a hangover when at home.

4. Experiencing cravings and urges, compulsions, to use a substance, especially in contexts where it's not relevant or appropriate, like constantly thinking about sparking up a joint while on the morning commute.

5. Similarly, your substance use prevents you from fulfilling your duties, at work, at school or at home. Important things are neglected because you're constantly seeking out, using, or recovering from your substance use.

6. Continuing to use a substance, even when those close to you are visibly upset and distressed by your doing so.

7. Similarly, not engaging with others, not going out, avoiding previously enjoyable social or recreational activities, because of substance use.

8. Continuing to use a substance, even when it puts you in danger, like having that third glass of wine and opting to drive home, even though you wrecked your last car and were lucky to escape without injury.

9. Related, persisting with substance use even though it's clearly making you unwell. Like smoking on top of a violent cough, or persisting with cocaine use even though it makes your existing paranoia even worse.

10. Finding you need more and more of a substance to achieve the desired effects. As in, once you got a pleasant buzz after three beers, but you now need eight, plus a few double whiskies, just to take the edge off.

11. Finally, feeling much worse if you *stop* taking a substance. If cutting off use gives you the shakes, sweats, a powerful sense of dread, or nausea, or anything that makes you feel terrible and further compels you to continue your consumption.

These are the eleven criteria for an addictive disorder, according to the DSM. The latest ICD has very similar criteria, but there are subtle divergences that reflect the different approaches of the DSM and the ICD, which we'll address later.

So, in summary, if your use of a substance is hard to control or stop, is more substantial than hoped, takes up most of your time, is maintained despite risks and dangers, makes you feel ill but you persist anyway, or makes you really ill if you try to stop, requires more and more intake to achieve the same enjoyable effects, and interferes with or disrupts your work, social life or relationships, then it's quite likely that you have an addiction.

Hopefully, you can now see why the claim that someone is addicted to their smartphone, or social media, is a bit much. They may be using them constantly, but if the device gets dropped and smashed, or the internet goes out for a few hours, they seldom start feeling physically unwell, or go to extreme, maybe even illegal lengths to log back in to Snapchat. Having said that, I've focused entirely on substance addiction so far, but that doesn't mean it's the only type of addiction. Again, we'll get to that soon.

I'd argue that all I've just talked about shows that addiction, like mostly everything else we've covered in this book, isn't a binary, yes-or-no thing, but more of a scale. And the DSM and mental health professionals seem to agree. If you show two or three of the eleven possible criteria for addiction within a twelve-month period, that's deemed a mild substance use disorder. Four or five, it's a moderate substance use disorder. Six or more, it's a severe substance use disorder.

Essentially, addiction is a very potent, very complex disorder. It shouldn't be thrown around, casually, by those who want to demonise and discredit things or behaviours they don't personally approve of. And yet, that happens all the time. Some people seem to really get off on it, to the point where they are unable to stop themselves from doing it and spend a lot of their time obsessing about it.

Anyone else spot the irony there?

Where in the brain does addiction happen?

Thus far, the focus has been on addiction caused by substances, meaning psychoactive chemicals, aka drugs.

The DSM lists ten separate classes of substances that can lead to addiction.

1. Alcohol, which we all know about.
2. Caffeine, another familiar friend.
3. Tobacco, or more typically 'smoking'.
4. Cannabis, or marijuana, weed, pot.
5. Hallucinogens, like LSD.
6. Opioids, like heroin and morphine, and numerous other painkillers, supposedly the big baddies of the drug world.
7. Sedatives, hypnotics, or anxiolytics like Valium, benzodiazepines, things discussed in the anxiety chapter.
8. Inhalants, things like huffing aerosols, sniffing glue, or amyl nitrate (widely known as poppers).
9. Stimulants, which run the gamut from amphetamines and cocaine to everyday caffeine.

That's nine separate categories of addictive substances. But I said there were ten. The final category is 'other or unknown substances'. Because there will still be plenty of chemicals out there that don't fall into those specific categories.

Like, antidepressants. They're definitely a psychoactive drug, but they're not included in this DSM list. Why? Because people rarely become addicted to them, due to the complex ways in which they work and operate and affect us. But *could* someone be addicted to them? Given how brains vary in how they respond to drugs, it can't be ruled out. So, if someone *were* addicted to antidepressants, they'd be deemed to have an addiction of the 'other' sort.

This point is a revealing one: the exact ways in which specific types of chemicals interact with our systems, and the effects they have on the brain, are frighteningly complex. Opiates like heroin, morphine, codeine and Vicodin* interact with the endorphin system in our brain. Endorphins are neurotransmitters that, among other things, suppress pain and induce euphoria, usually at times of great physical stress.[3] People who run marathons or do other lengthy, strenuous exercise describe the 'runner's high', where they experience a great euphoric rush as their running continues. It's when your brain realises your body is experiencing significant physical stress and hardship and so pumps you full of endorphins to take the pain away, make you feel good, and allow you to better deal with whatever's supposedly

---

* A combination of acetaminophen and hydrocodone, made famous by the aforementioned TV show House M.D., where the eponymous lead character was addicted to Vicodin.

causing this physical misery.* Opiates essentially hijack this system, stimulating the relevant receptors on the relevant neurons, causing intense pleasure. And subsequent addiction.

With alcohol, for many years it was believed its effects were due to how the ethanol molecule – the stuff in booze that actually gets you drunk – is so small that it can pass through the membranes of neurons with no trouble. If there's ethanol in your body, keeping it out of cells is like trying to carry water in a wicker basket. Once it's inside neurons, ethanol disrupts the neuronal workings, temporarily throwing out the delicate chemical processes that keep everything running smoothly. And so, we get drunk.

However, more modern data suggest that alcohol also seems to boost the GABA system particularly,[4] meaning more neurological systems get suppressed, like our coordination, speech, rational thinking, and more. Benzodiazepines also boost the GABA system, as we saw. And these are very relaxing, very enjoyable, very addictive.

Tobacco, specifically nicotine, interacts with acetylcholine receptors in the frontal regions of the brain. Cocaine triggers a range of dopamine receptors. Caffeine works on the calcium channels of certain neurons, increasing activity. And so on, and so on. It's a very rich tapestry. It would require many volumes of other books to explain the way certain chemicals affect our brains, with any degree of thoroughness.

However, despite all this variety, there does seem to be one

* I can't personally confirm this, as I don't think I've run 26 miles thus far, in my life. But I'm reliably informed it's a thing.

brain region underpinning most, if not *all* cases of addiction. Remember how in the previous chapter, we discussed the threat detection system? That circuit in your brain that scans for and reacts to anything deemed hazardous or dangerous, causing us to get scared and stressed in response? Well, that's not the only mechanism like this in the brain. In this case, there's the reward pathway.

The reward pathway is a surprisingly small circuit, found down in the deeper, central regions of our brain.[5] There are two basic parts. There's the nucleus accumbens, and this connects to the ventral tegmental area. We covered the ventral tegmental area earlier, in the depression chapter; it's an integral part of our ability to feel good, or nice. Essentially, the nucleus accumbens is fed information about everything going on in the brain. If it recognises anything as being good, beneficial or generally positive, it sends signals direct to the ventral tegmental area. This, via complex connections to our most basic systems in the brainstem and beyond, causes us to experience pleasure. The sensation of pleasure, *reward*, comes from this pathway. It's sometimes called the mesolimbic reward pathway. And it's sometimes called the dopaminergic reward pathway, because dopamine, another monoamine transmitter, is the neurotransmitter this pathway uses to do its job, to give us the sensation of pleasure at the most fundamental level.

As mentioned earlier, you may have heard dopamine called the pleasure chemical, or the happy chemical – and this is why. But this idea that dopamine is the chemical responsible for pleasure, and *only* that – so boosting dopamine levels is all you need for pleasure, to be happy – is laughably simplistic.

If you want to boost dopamine levels throughout your brain, quickly and easily, get hold of some levodopa, the default drug used for patients with Parkinson's disease.[6] Parkinson's disease is caused by the gradual degradation of the substantia nigra, involved in movement and mood control, and other things. This region also uses dopamine. Its loss means less dopamine is being sent to necessary areas, resulting in Parkinson's disease symptoms. Levodopa boosts dopamine levels throughout the brain, so this loss is compensated for.

However, if increasing dopamine automatically caused pleasure and happiness, people with Parkinson's should be in a constant state of bliss, and levodopa should be the most popular drug on the planet. But they aren't, and it isn't. In truth, the activation of the reward pathway is very complex and variable. It evolved to encourage us and reward us for things that are beneficial in some way, so we remember them better and want to keep doing them. However, there is an eye-wateringly vast range of things that can be deemed beneficial, from an intensely pleasurable sexual experience to a successful social encounter, to a mere glass of water if we're hot and thirsty. Activation of the reward pathway is tied to activity in countless other areas of the brain, and the reward pathway in turn sends out many connections and signals to other essential brain regions, especially those involved in thinking, motivation and emotion.

The result of this is that things we derive pleasure from, that make us happy, play a huge role in how we think, how

254

we behave, the decisions we make, and more, right down at the neurological level. How could they not?

But you can have *too much* of a good thing. Like with the threat detection pathway, the human brain has evolved a number of traits and behaviours that can cause hassle and confusion for the long-established, pleasure-inducing reward pathway, and the sophisticated balance it has with other important brain processes.

And that's without introducing foreign substances into our body, which activate the reward pathway more or less directly, skipping the sophisticated checks and balances our brain has built up over the millennia. That, with varying degrees of directness, is what addictive substances do: activate the reward pathway, when it otherwise *wouldn't* be activated. There are many ways of achieving this activation, of course.

That's how you can have addiction to stimulants *and* sedatives. They have exactly the opposite effects on us – how can both be equally addictive?! But they are. Stimulants may interact with relevant receptors to trigger the reward pathway directly, causing increased activity and pleasure, while sedatives may shut down certain brain regions that are *suppressing* the reward pathway, or increasing concern and stress, leading to elevated levels of reward-pathway activity, and therefore pleasure. That, in a nutshell, is why different substances result in the same condition, i.e. addiction. They're all affecting the same part of the brain, the reward pathway, but in different ways and via different means.

It's like those old eighties race movies, such as *The Cannonball Run*, where a bunch of whacky characters race across the country for a grand prize. They use different routes, different vehicles, have different adventures on the way, but eventually all end up in the same place. Substance abuse and addiction is sort of like that, regarding how it works in the brain. Although, unlike a screwball eighties comedy, you can't just turn addiction off and wonder what on earth was going on there. No, the effects are just getting started. And they're very rarely amusing.

The impact of addiction: the stadium in the brain

I keep bringing up certain things about the brain again and again. But it's because these things are very important in the context of mental health. And one of these is how flexible, how plastic, the brain is. It doesn't just sit there and passively absorb what's going on; it adapts, it changes, it anticipates and adjusts and responds. When it can't do that so much, we get depression – at least, according to modern evidence. So, the brain being unable to change and adapt is a bad thing.

But, conversely (and confusingly), the brain being *able* to adapt can be a bad thing too. We saw that in the last chapter, where the brain adapted to constant activity from the amygdala and stress system, altering important neurological processes in unhelpful ways. In essence, anxiety problems arise when our brains adapt to things that shouldn't be happening, namely excessive activity in the threat and stress systems. You get the same thing in addiction. The reward pathway is being stimulated to a degree far beyond what the brain is set up to deal with. So, it adapts and changes, so it *can* deal with it.

Unfortunately, this excess activity is caused by an external agent, usually the drug being abused. So, you have lasting changes taking place in your brain, in response to something that isn't always present in the brain, that must be administered from the outside. This can be very bad. Here's an analogy to explain how and why.

Imagine a small town, with a small population. A perfectly normal, self-sustaining town. Then, for some reason, a huge stadium is built right in the middle of it, where the town hall used to be. A stadium that regularly hosts major football matches, concerts by the most popular bands, and other massive events.

This would mean that, all of a sudden, tens of thousands of people descend upon the town, to attend the stadium.

Initially, the town is going to be seriously overwhelmed. This can be a positive thing: every hotel, hostel and Airbnb is booked. Every bar, restaurant and café is at capacity, with queues out the door. Every shop is sold out. All the taxis and buses are full, for hours on end. The town's economy gets a flood of new money, so everyone is better off.

But the town doesn't get much done while the stadium is in use. There's not enough transport, not enough food and drink stockpiled, insufficient police and security to keep everyone and everything under control. The road system can't cope. A lot of things grind to a halt. This is bad, and unsustainable. So, logically, the town gradually changes, to accommodate the regular stadium crowds. More roads are built, more hotels and bars and shops spring up, more police and security are employed.

257

The thing is, though, if this continues for long enough, eventually much of the town will be dedicated to catering for visitors to the stadium. Rather than being enriched but overwhelmed by stadium crowds, the town now depends on them; they're vital for sustaining this new set-up. What was once exceptional is now the norm, the baseline.

And then, the stadium vanishes. One morning it's just gone. There's only the old town hall again, which holds a couple of hundred people at most. Maybe that was enough once. But it's not now. The town hall is now surrounded by an enlarged community that *needs* crowds of tens of thousands, to keep functioning normally. So, they can either frantically build a new stadium, to keep the crowds coming. Or they can go back to the old set-up, enduring a lot of pain and hardship along the way as businesses collapse and people become destitute.

An elaborate, evocative image, perhaps. But a useful one. The town is a standard brain, the town hall is the normal reward pathway, the appearance of the stadium is the first hit of a powerful, pleasurable drug. If the stadium appeared one day and disappeared the next, perhaps everything would be OK. The town would remember that one intense night with a mix of fondness, confusion and alarm, but it would otherwise carry on as normal. Similarly, people who dabble in narcotics and illicit substances, but don't use them persistently, often talk about their 'experimentation phase', or their wild nights. But these aren't things that affect them now.

But if the stadium remains, if you keep using a drug, the town changes and adapts to accommodate it. Likewise, your brain remodels itself to adapt to the drug, to incorporate its constant presence. So much so, that eventually the *absence* of the drug causes more problems than its presence.

This is expressed via several changes in the very structure of the brain, resulting from excessive activity in the reward pathway, and these underlie many of the classic properties of an addictive disorder.

Getting used to tolerance

One of the more familiar symptoms of addiction is tolerance, where the same dose of a drug affects you less and less over time. So, the dose must be increased, to achieve the same level of pleasurable effects. Those pleasurable effects are the whole point of taking the drug, after all.

This tolerance can happen surprisingly quickly. Some call crack cocaine 'the broken promise', because the first high it provides is incredibly intense and pleasurable. But no subsequent high will ever feel as good, because you (or more specifically, your brain's processes) adapt to it rapidly. This can mean users are more likely to persist with the drug, trying to recapture that first feeling. Sadly, they can't. A broken promise.

Remember, just like the stadium in the town example, while a potent drug might be incredibly pleasurable, it's also very overwhelming. That's why when someone is under the influence of a potent narcotic, you don't let them do anything important or risky, like drive a car, or perform surgery. A powerful drug may be enjoyable, but it stops the brain from doing much, from functioning right. So, fundamental processes kick in immediately, to adapt, to stop this happening again.

There are numerous mechanisms at work.[7] The reward pathway, running on dopamine, may see increased numbers of dopamine receptors in the component neurons, meaning more dopamine, more stimulation, is required to achieve standard levels of activity and response. Or, existing receptors may become desensitised, so they don't respond as powerfully, as enthusiastically, to standard stimulation. Or, more neurons get involved in the circuit governing this particular response, so can reduce or suppress the initially excessive stimulus.

Overall, it usually means more dopamine, more activity, is required in the reward pathway to trigger a pleasure response. The first experience of the drug caught the reward pathway by surprise, and it starts essentially cladding itself in armour so that doesn't happen again so easily. Hence, next time the drug appears it still causes a response, but not such a strong one. So, to get the same response, you need more of the drug to get the desired reaction from the reward pathway. Which then responds by getting more defensive, more desensitised, and a sort of drug/pleasure arms race begins.

And it's not just the brain. The body isn't being idle during all this. Drugs must be ingested, inhaled or injected, to get to the brain. Whichever it is, the relevant body parts and tissues recognise that this substance isn't meant to be there, so they adapt too, stepping up their breakdown and clearance processes. So, successive doses of a drug are often broken down and booted out more quickly, giving them less time and opportunity to have an effect. The body and brain effectively learn from the presence of a drug, and work to cancel it out. So, more of the drug is needed each time, to keep the pleasurable effects intact.

Unfortunately, the parts of the brain being changed by the drug aren't parts that are used exclusively by drugs, like some hitherto unused VIP lounge. No, by becoming less responsive to drug stimulation, the reward pathway is also less responsive to *everything else*. Therefore, previously enjoyable things, such as fun social encounters and hobbies and decent food, become less pleasurable, of less importance, for those experiencing an addiction. It's no wonder they often lose interest in their more everyday routines and pastimes; their brain may have adapted to the point where increased doses of the drug are the only thing that *can* cause pleasure, so they pursue it even more enthusiastically.

Tolerance also causes problems because, while the reward pathway is the brain region you want the drug to affect, it's not the *only* bit that will be affected. Remember how taking antidepressants and similar medications means they're present throughout body and brain, so have multiple effects in multiple areas? The exact same is true for recreational drugs (most of which started out as medicines in the first place), and if you increase the dose of a drug because you've grown tolerant, you're going to increase the side effects too. And in too-high doses, drugs can be fatal. Too much alcohol can suppress the respiratory mechanisms that control your breathing. Heroin and other opiates can wreak havoc on the functioning of the heart, and so on. Such things are very difficult to recover from. Can the brain become so tolerant to a drug that using it becomes a precarious balance between pleasure and death? It's an extreme outcome, but sure. Can't rule it out.

You'd think that surely everybody, no matter how far into their drug habit, would pull back from the brink before things got that serious? Before it meant their own death? That's the only logical option.

This would be the case, if an addiction spared your brain's ability to think logically. But obviously, it doesn't.

How your addiction rules your thinking

You may look at someone with a severe addiction and think: why on earth would they keep at it? They're driving away everyone close to them. They're seriously damaging their health and well-being. They're sacrificing everything they've worked for. They're being shunned by society at large, risking their own lives and the wrath of the law. All just to feed a drug habit? For a few moments of pleasure? It doesn't make sense.

Obviously, not every addiction is so extreme. Most aren't. But the mainstream portrayal of addiction is often along these lines. Maybe it's because the most high-profile addicts are invariably celebrities, those who achieve huge fame and acclaim, only to lose it all, and often their own lives, thanks to drug addiction. How can that possibly make sense to anyone? Admittedly, life as a major star no doubt has many complications and variables that affect how you make decisions. I wouldn't know.

Even without the distorting shell of fame, evidence shows that repeated, chronic drug use and addiction alters how you think. So, what may seem like a no-brainer decision to you can seem like the exact opposite to someone in the grip of addiction. It is deemed a mental disorder, after all, so disruption of thinking and cognition is undoubtedly a big part of it.[8]

We're often told to 'follow your dreams', 'do what you love', 'treat yourself', and so on. The things we like and derive pleasure and satisfaction from play a big role in determining how we think, act and plan, over both the short and long term. This is facilitated by connections between our prefrontal cortex, our thinking and planning and rationalisation areas, and the reward pathway. Because how often do you think about doing something because you feel, or know, that you'll enjoy it?

Similarly, frontal regions of the brain, prefrontal cortex included, comprise a complex network that gives rise to and processes motivation. Some label it goal-directed behaviour. It's ostensibly our ability to recognise a goal, which guides us to think and act in ways that allow us to achieve it. Again, the reward system is a key component here. Even if the goal itself isn't objectively pleasurable, like spending an hour at the gym, the successful completion of a goal, of doing something arduous that gets us closer to our desired end-state, can be quite rewarding. Countless people report satisfaction and contentment after 'an honest day's work', as they put it. This is a big part of that.

Indeed, we often only have certain goals and ideals in the first place because we've learned they're rewarding in some way. The enjoyment of team interaction and victory can spur someone's desire to be a professional footballer. The thrilling childhood experience of being applauded for singing a song in a school play can lead to dreams of musical stardom. The reward and pleasure parts of the brain also support our ability to learn, in the most basic, fundamental ways. At the most simple, neurological level, connections are made between something happening, and how good or bad the outcome of it was.

If we do a thing and something bad happens, we avoid doing it again. If we do a thing and nothing happens, we don't associate any outcome to it. If we do a thing and something rewarding happens, we experience pleasure, so we learn that this is a good thing, and are inclined to seek it out and do it again. Our bulky brains are obviously capable of far more sophisticated learning processes than this, but much of our thinking and learning is still heavily influenced by these basic principles, the ones of associative learning and conditioning,[9] the same thing demonstrated by Pavlov's famous dogs. Overall, it's always easier to learn and remember things we enjoy, as opposed to things we're indifferent to.

The main point of all this is to emphasise that the reward pathway is heavily involved in the mechanisms underlying motivation, planning, thinking, and more. We previously saw that the amygdala is similarly integrated in many of our thinking and reasoning processes, so an overactive amygdala can give everything we experience a stressful, anxiety-inducing slant. A similar thing comes about via the reward pathway. When it's overactive, overstimulated by substances, this brings about changes. But not just in that pathway; it affects many of the things it's linked to as well, like those areas charged with thinking, motivation, and more.

One of the more distressing hallmarks of addiction is how the addicted individual seems to prioritise their addiction over all other needs and drives. They seem to care much less, or not at all, for friends and family, for looking after their health and well-being, or even their own safety. At the extremes, addiction even seems to cause a loss of concern for basic hygiene and obeying social, or even legal, norms.

This is another source of intense stigma, of course. We've been over how a mental health problem can damage relationships, because of the effect it can have on a person's behaviour, and compliance with expected social norms. Well, what about an affliction that causes you to disregard anyone and everyone, and even your own health? Forming a negative opinion of such a person would be pretty much automatic, even though their thinking and motivation has been disrupted in ways they're probably not aware of.

To make it clearer, being addicted to a substance genuinely alters how you think and act regarding it. It's not just a failure of self-control, shameless indulgence, or flawed priorities, as many seem to think. It's more that use of the drug means the parts of the brain responsible for self-control, recognising risks and hazards and setting priorities have been genuinely altered, co-opted even, so that acquisition of the drug takes precedence over everything else.[10] And because the very processes underlying thinking and motivation have been altered, a genuine addict may find it difficult even to recognise that their behaviour and thinking is harmful, to themselves or others.

It's not automatically a sense of shame, guilt or fear that causes people to deny or downplay their addictions. Those things are relevant, no doubt, but in many cases, the internal workings of their brain have adapted to the presence of a drug in ways that make them less able to recognise that anything is amiss, or to downplay or minimise it if they do – because so much of the brain is geared towards self-preservation, shielding ego, identity, beliefs and worldview from change and disruption. And if your addiction becomes part of these things, your brain will become wired to instinctively defend that too.

This isn't to say that an addicted person *can't* think, that they're intellectually stunted in some way. Far from it. Most addicts retain their normal faculties in every other area. Indeed, many people find their creativity and intellect enhanced while under the influence. But there's a sort of blind spot or *cognitive filter* in place when it comes to analysing their drug habit and coming to realistic conclusions. For this reason, getting someone to even admit they have an addiction is a stressful process. Getting them to actually do something about it is considerably more so again.

And speaking of stressful . . .

The serious stress of quitting

As with many things described thus far, while some addicted individuals may be genuinely unable to think about their addiction rationally, that's a relatively extreme manifestation. Because, when you think about it, countless addicts at least *attempt* to quit. That's even one of the criteria for addiction: unsuccessful attempts to quit. Regardless of whether they succeed, rational thought and self-awareness are clearly still something an addict is capable of, even if they're compromised. They can still recognise that there's a problem, decide they need to do something about it, and be motivated enough to make the effort.

So, why is giving up still so difficult? If it's just a matter of recognising a problem and avoiding the cause of it, why do so many people struggle? Why is rehab such a prolonged process? Why is relapse so common? A big part of it is withdrawal, where if an addict stops taking their drug, they experience *deeply* unpleasant reactions.

Why?

One problem is all those neurological changes that have occurred in an addicted brain; they don't instantly disappear once the drug is removed. The town around the stadium doesn't go right back to normal just because the stadium vanishes. If you remove a drug from an addicted brain, particularly if you do so abruptly, you're basically taking a very complex system and ripping out a key part of it, like yanking the spark plugs out of a car engine while you're driving on the motorway.

But it's not just a case of brain regions that depend on drug-induced activity now being denied them and struggling to function. Recent research has revealed something else that makes the whole thing worse again. We've seen many times that the brain has numerous checks and balances in place. We have the *approach* and *avoid* motivation systems. We have excitatory glutamate neurons that increase activity, and GABA neurons that suppress it. We have the amygdala to make us wary of threats, and the prefrontal cortex that makes us stop worrying. And now it seems that as well as a reward system, we have an *anti*-reward system.

The available data suggest this anti-reward system incorporates a lot of the stress system, like parts of the amygdala and stria terminalis. It also uses chemicals like corticotrophin-releasing factor and dynorphin, which have been shown to be abnormally high in those with depression, or in suicide victims. These chemicals have multiple roles, but overall seem to induce a state of dysphoria, the opposite of euphoria. Basically, the anti-reward system makes us experience discomfort and distress.

Here's the tricky part: evidence suggests that when we experience something pleasurable, it causes significant activity in the reward pathway, as we know, but also mild activity in the anti-reward pathway.

This could be just to keep the anti-reward pathway active, keeping something ticking over when it's not in use, so it's ready to go when needed. But it's more likely that it's to do with balance. We've had the reward pathways in our brain for a very long time, and as we've seen, too much reward pathway activity is a bad thing. It would make sense, there-fore, for the brain to have something in place to prevent us from losing ourselves, to counteract something that causes excess pleasure. Research suggests that activity in the anti-reward pathway goes up as activity in our reward pathway goes down.

It's a clever system, and one I bet we've all experienced to some extent. Have you ever liked a food so much you've gorged yourself on it? Or fallen so in love with a song you listened to it on repeat for days on end? If you do that, it's fun. At first. But soon you grow sick of your favoured thing. The thought of eating more of that stuff becomes distressing. That song makes you grit your teeth rather than tap your feet. If it was just a case of your reward pathway adapting to them, you'd presumably not react to them at all. But you're not just unresponsive to your previously beloved thing, you're actively repelled by it. This suggests that your anti-reward system now has the upper hand. It's a neat set-up, really. It's like a fail-safe, to prevent us from being consumed by our desire to indulge.

At least, that's what's meant to happen in normal brains. But remember, drugs *aren't* a normal aspect of brains. They don't induce pleasure via our inbuilt systems, like food or music do. They essentially jump the queue and stimulate the reward system directly,* so we don't become so readily re-pulsed by or tired of them. They also push things, namely activity in the reward system, beyond normal limits. And the anti-reward system is constantly trying to catch up.

---

* Or at least 'artificially', in a sense.

So, as well as an extremely unresponsive reward system, drugs simultaneously gift you with a supercharged anti-reward system. And remember what I said about the reward pathway not being just for the drug, but for everything pleasurable? The same applies to the anti-reward pathway; it responds to pretty much everything. The thinking is that the anti-reward pathway, substantially enhanced by chronic drug use, overreacts to everything, because the usual base-line activity and precise balances are totally out of whack. And this causes considerably more distress, displeasure and discomfort in the addicted brain, in response to even minor stresses and hassles.

Ask any long-term drug addict, they'll say the days of taking the drug to feel good are long gone. Now, they take it solely so they can feel *normal*. The internal balance of their brain needs a minimum dose of the drug to induce enough activity in the reward pathway to cancel out the hugely enhanced anti-reward activity. That's why withdrawal is a thing. It's why going cold turkey is such an ordeal. It doesn't just mean an absence of drug-induced pleasure, it's more a presence of major discomfort and distress, thanks to a bloated anti-reward system making you incredibly sensitive to anything unpleasant.

The previous anxiety chapter showed how bad things get when the brain's stress system is even mildly overactive. A long-term addict's stress system, of which the anti-reward system is a big part, is substantially overactive. On top of this, their reward system, the part that allows pleasure and cancels out pain and stress, is as unresponsive as possible, like the calluses on a clumsy carpenter's thumb. Overall, it means cold turkey, undergoing extreme withdrawal, quickly provides all the worst effects of serious stress and pain, and literally nothing can make them feel better, because the part of their brain that allows them to feel better is barely responsive. Apart from their usual drug. Hence, cold turkey is such a deeply unpleasant experience. In extreme cases, it can be so severe it causes injuries, or even death.[11]

This also helps explain why relapse is so common, why staying clean is so difficult for many. Those changes that have occurred in the brain, they never *entirely* go away. All those circuits that learned that a certain drug means pleasure or relief, all that bulking up of the stress system, that's still there. They might be diminished, toned down, or dormant, but as adaptive as the brain can be, it often doesn't get rid of them entirely. These changes are the result of persistent use of powerful drugs, but a *lack* of something doesn't really have the same impact as a *presence* of something. Having your house burn down once will make you very vigilant and wary of fires. The countless times your house doesn't burn down afterwards won't really change that.

My point is, the brain changes that result from long-term addiction – they linger. It doesn't take much to set them off again. The modifications of the thinking and planning regions mean it's hard for an addict not to think of their addiction. The anti-reward system enhancement means a stress response is more potent, so anything stressful happening in their lives (a common occurrence for recovering addicts) hits them a lot harder, making them more desperate to put a stop to it. And if the only thing that you know can do that is your drug of choice? Well . . .

Admittedly, all of this is based on the extreme end of the addiction spectrum. We're talking constant use of the most powerful narcotics, like heroin. Not every drug is this potent or goes this far. But that doesn't mean they're easy to quit. How many people try, and fail, to give up smoking? Sure, cigarettes are relatively mild in terms of drug potency, but smoking still causes changes in your fundamental neurological workings, which can be hard to power through.

And if using a drug is deemed 'not so bad', it means the consequences of keeping going, and not quitting, aren't so bad either. So, there's less incentive, less motivation, to quit smoking, particularly if you're experiencing a lot of stress. It varies from drug to drug, obviously. But an addiction is an addiction, the underlying mechanics are still basically the same.

And here's the weird thing: sometimes addiction can happen without a drug being involved at all.

Addicted to behaviours, not just drugs

Heroin addiction is often treated with methadone. It's another opiate drug, but its different chemical properties mean it tackles the worst of heroin withdrawal symptoms without maintaining the addiction. It's sort of a halfway house on the road to sobriety, to get someone over the worst of withdrawal, so they can regain self-control and avoid the drug without countless parts of their brain and body screaming in pain.

People react to methadone differently – an effective course can take as little as one month to as many as six – but it seems to do the job. Except, there are often weird complications and problems that occur.

For example, another key difference between heroin and methadone is how it's taken. The more serious heroin users inject it. By contrast, methadone is taken orally; it's swallowed, often in the form of a bright green liquid.* Technically, this shouldn't be an issue; through the mouth or through the veins, if the chemical effect on the brain is the same, what does it matter?

Unfortunately, humans aren't that simple. There are reports of addicts who take their methadone, but don't swallow it. Instead, they actually spit it into a syringe and inject it. It's gross, dangerously unhygienic, and makes the drug less effective. So, why do that?

It's another instance where the human brain is *too* powerful, because it doesn't just recognise the basic chemical effect of a drug, it also encodes all the detail and methods and behaviours of taking the drug. Long story short, if you regularly inject a drug, your brain learns that *injecting is pleasurable*, so it becomes a pleasurable act in itself. You go from injecting to swallowing a drug, you're being short-changed as far as your brain's concerned. This can be the difference between a treatment working, or not. Remember, the possibility of something bad happening literally causes a stress response that affects us physically. And the same is

* It looks a lot like a fairy-tale potion, which may be a good or bad thing.

true here; thinking that something is genuinely pleasurable often makes it so.

It's not just injecting heroin. 'Vaping' with e-cigarettes is very popular now and seems to have had more luck than nicotine gum, or patches, with regards to getting people off cigarettes (within reason).[12] Why? One explanation is that putting something in your mouth and inhaling is far closer to the act of smoking, something your brain strongly associates with a nicotine hit. So, inhaling satisfies the nicotine craving, in ways an inert patch on the arm won't.

And many casual smokers report that they're mostly fine with not smoking, but can't resist lighting up when they're drinking. True, alcohol lowers inhibitions, so the ability to resist the urge to smoke is weakened, and they succumb. Over time, a strong association between drinking and nicotine would develop and enhance the craving, the expectation, for a cigarette in the presence of alcohol.

However, these are all behaviours that are part of the drug-taking routine, or ritual, if you prefer. But here's the question: can behaviours be addictive all by themselves, without an outside chemical substance entering the equation? Would our brain's complexity mean the pleasure-producing part of the brain can be pushed too far, giving rise to the effects of addiction, by certain stimulating actions or behaviours?

Apparently so. But here, the evidence base is a lot murkier.

When the DSM-4 updated to the DSM-5, there was now a new entry in the substance-related and addictive disorders category: gambling addiction.[13] The evidence had been reviewed and it was deemed that, while it involved no psychoactive substances, gambling addiction meets enough of the conditions to be classed alongside the more well-known drug addictions, as a genuine addictive disorder. Gambling addicts regularly try to stop, but can't. They gamble way more than they can afford. They lose relationships and jobs and give up social lives to feed their addiction. They deny that they have a problem, even if it's blatant. And so on. So sure, gambling addiction is an addictive disorder. Why wouldn't it be?

That's a good question. And why just gambling? Aren't there many other behaviours that are clearly addictive? Possibly. But again, it's not so straightforward. When it comes to behavioural issues, there are a lot of other ways to define or describe them without invoking full-blown addiction.

Previously, gambling was deemed an 'impulse control disorder'. A different type of mental health problem. When you know that a certain behaviour will be pleasurable, you are instinctively, impulsively, driven to do it. But if this behaviour or action, despite being pleasurable, would probably, or definitely, have negative consequences, you are aware that you shouldn't do it, so you stop yourself.

Most people can weigh up the pros and cons and restrain themselves from obeying this enjoyable but risky impulse. Sure, it would be pleasurable to have sex with this woman, but I'm married, and so is she, to my best friend. It would be an enjoyable experience, but one that would ruin all our lives, so I won't. Or, it would be nice to have more money, so I could take that person's unattended wallet. But I'd be breaking the law, with all the negative consequences that can lead to. And the innocent owner of the wallet would be harmed by my actions, so I won't do it.

It's yet another example, if you like, of the general structure and set-up of our brains. Older, simpler systems provoke a quick, unthinking reaction. But our newer, smarter thought processes step in and put the brakes on, with their greater awareness of long-term consequences. The older, simpler subconscious processes occur very quickly, so we still experience the impulse to do something gratifying without even thinking about it. Thankfully, our smarter processes are quick and powerful enough to stop us from acting on the impulse. They can't stop the impulse outright, but they can stop it dictating our behaviour. They provide restraint.

But if you have an impulse control disorder, you often lack this restraint, this ability to say 'I won't.' You may well possess the awareness that something will be bad, but are unable to stop yourself from doing it anyway. Impulse control issues also have a distinct, well-defined arc, where the individual experiences an impulse, growing tension as the impulse isn't acted on, pleasure when the impulse *is* acted on, relief from the removal of the tension, and finally guilt, or shame. The last one may not occur, but it may also be severe.

While there is some considerable overlap, this *isn't* the same as addiction.[14] An impulse control disorder is qualitatively different, in many ways. Impulse control disorders, for example, don't seem to feature the lack of recognition that there's a problem, something common in addiction. And impulse control disorder doesn't seem to come with the deprioritising of other important facets of the individual's life;

they don't seem to care less about work and relationships – guilt and shame wouldn't be so common for them if they did. Impulse control disorders also don't seem to feature the sort of tolerance and withdrawal that's common in many addictions.

As stated, though, there's a great deal of overlap between addiction and impulse control disorder. A lack of impulse control undoubtedly leads to you being more likely to try drugs or illicit activities in the first place, therefore dramatically raising the odds of you becoming addicted. Conversely, some report that if you're addicted to something already, you have poorer impulse control – which makes sense, given how your brain's self-control processes have been compromised, as mentioned.

But still, it's important, for all the reasons discussed earlier, to be as clear as possible when it comes to diagnosing someone. Therefore, it's necessary to distinguish between impulse control disorders and addictions.

Not that this is easy. It gets even more confusing when you introduce the cultural and societal aspects too. For instance, the term sex addiction is a common one, but cases of excessive sexual behaviour, or hypersexuality, are far more likely to be deemed impulse control disorders.[15] The evidence that you can be genuinely addicted to sex, that you cannot function without it and that obtaining it consumes your life, is still not conclusive.

But this is a particularly tricky one, as the typical sources of addiction, things like alcohol, opiates and nicotine, are external agents, strangers to our bodily systems. We know that the correct amount of heroin someone should be injecting is zero heroin. But a mature human wanting sex? That's meant to happen. So where do you draw the line between normal human sex drive and a clinical disorder? Because it's a fundamental human drive, who's to say how much sex is too much? We all have our personal preferences, but what you want and what the next person wants regarding sex can vary wildly. And there are so many stifling cultural expectations confusing matters too. Remember in the first chapter we spoke of nymphomania, because women wanting a lot of sex was deemed a mental disorder for a worryingly long time, rather than a standard expression of human variability?

Admittedly, there are many types of problematic sexual behaviour recognised by the mental health fields, like hypersexuality, where people want and pursue sex way beyond reasonable expectations, or limits, to the extent that it harms their lifestyle and situation. But in many other cases, the uncertainty around what counts as genuinely unhealthy sexual behaviour is a constant problem.

Technology is another thing that's confusing matters. Smartphone and internet addiction are also terms that are regularly thrown around in the media, but again, the evidence behind such claims is far less certain. An extensive study published in 2018 in the *Journal of Behavioural Addictions* concluded that, despite them regularly being described as such, there's no clear evidence that smartphones are actually addictive,[16] in the strictest sense of the word. This doesn't mean they're totally harmless, or can't be overused, or won't lead to negative changes in behaviour. It's just that these don't meet the threshold for an addiction diagnosis. The authors suggest adopting new terms, such as 'problematic use' or 'maladaptive behaviours', to describe excessive, disruptive smartphone use.

Could it be said that smartphones lead to impulse control disorders, though? It seems that it could, given how often people check their phones for no discernible reason. But do they experience the urge, the tension, the pleasure, and the guilt when checking their phone? Most would say no, it's a far more innocuous, everyday occurrence. Maybe smartphones do indeed need their own original terms to describe the behaviour issues they lead to.

Similarly, is internet addiction a thing? Should it be considered a genuine mental health issue? You might think so. Countless people spend every waking hour online, no matter what it does for their health or social lives. How could they *not* be addicted? The problem with that argument is, what do the words 'online' or 'internet' *mean* here? They're far broader than is clinically useful. For example, what if someone spends all their time online chatting to friends, and playing games as part of a group? Far from severing relationships, they're cultivating them. They're not rejecting their pastimes, they're pursuing them. That's the exact opposite of what you'd expect from an addiction. This is possible because you can be constantly online *and* have a rich social life, and hobbies. Technology has progressed to the point where that's an option. This makes diagnosing based on strict criteria even trickier.

Or, what if someone's constantly playing online roulette? Is that an internet addiction, or a gambling addiction? The internet may be the conduit it's delivered by, but it's the gambling that's the issue. If they did the same thing in a casino, would we call that a building addiction? No.

But could you argue that it's an impulse control disorder? Maybe, but even then, it's questionable, because impulse control disorders seem contingent on being unable to stop yourself doing something, despite the negative consequences. But simply 'being online' doesn't really have any disastrous outcomes 99 per cent of the time. It's a fairly neutral experience. And because of Wi-Fi and technology being as omnipresent as it is now, most people are constantly online in some shape or form.

Once again, we have the problem of trying to build reliable, rigorous diagnostic criteria on ever-shifting cultural sands.

Does looking at it in terms of the brain offer any clarity or reliability? Possibly. There are numerous neurological features that at least offer some insight. For instance, you don't tend to have the co-opting of the reward pathway in impulse control disorders that you would expect with addiction. Adaptation and tolerance in an impulse control disorder also seem to be a more gradual, smaller-scale affair, if they happen at all. And there are indeed specific brain regions tied to impulse control, and if they show atypical activity, it helps to determine if it's really a disorder that an individual is dealing with. Poor sexual inhibition is often associated with reduced activity in the orbitofrontal cortex, part of the frontal lobe strongly linked to self-control and impulse regulation.

Correspondingly, increased activity in the orbitofrontal cortex has been observed in sexual dysfunctions, in those who struggle to become aroused or perform sexually. That's what you'd expect if the part of your brain that says 'No, don't do that' was overactive. If you were looking for where in the brain a problem with impulse control could stem from, you could do much worse than the orbitofrontal cortex. Again, though, impulse control disorders and addiction may be distinct things on paper, but they undeniably do feed into each other in complex ways. Like anxiety and depression do, in a sense.

Another type of behavioural disorder that's often mistaken for addiction is compulsive disorders, the most famous being obsessive-compulsive disorder, OCD. Being unable to stop yourself doing something that serves no purpose and is often detrimental to your life and situation: that describes addiction. It also describes OCD. But again, there are key differences. As with impulse control disorders, someone with a compulsion problem remains aware that their behaviour and drives are not great, but is mostly helpless to stop them. Meanwhile, those with addictions regularly deny they have a problem, even to themselves.

Also, one particularly important difference is that, in contrast to both addictions and impulse control disorders, the compulsion is rarely something *pleasurable*. Biting your nails, washing your hands, checking your door three dozen times before leaving your house: there's no buzz or euphoria or pleasure for those compelled to do these things, it just feels wrong if they're not done. The only real positive is the relief from having done them. Addictions, meanwhile, invariably begin with something that causes pleasure, and are

281

often cemented by repeated efforts to re-experience it. That's also how impulse control and compulsions differ; the impulse is to do something that is pleasurable in the short term, although a bad idea overall, while the compulsion is usually to do something atypical that doesn't really have any immediate reward.

There is also now a substantial body of evidence that shows the neurological underpinnings of OCD and other compulsive disorders are markedly different from what's seen in addiction, or impulse control disorders. Compulsive disorders do seem to have a lot more to do with problems in communication between key brain regions, like the striatum and thalamus, and other systems that control initiation and cessation of behaviours and actions. There have also been studies that show flaws in the white matter tracts of the compulsive brain. White matter is basically the conduits and cables of the brain that link everything up, so this communication issue is further supported by this. It basically seems like the signals that say 'Stop' or 'Don't' are blocked or obscured in a compulsive brain, so they end up constantly doing things they've no real reason to do.

In truth, the data suggest that most compulsive individuals *don't* do the whole obsessive cleaning or repetitive actions thing, which is how OCD is normally portrayed and thought of. Instead, most people are afflicted with compulsive thought, in that they can't stop thinking about, dwelling on, a random thought or unusual idea, and this can hamper their normal cognitive functioning in a variety of ways. We all of us have random, weird thoughts, all the time. Most of us can dismiss these idle fantasies and bizarre notions as just fleeting contemplations. People with compulsive disorders seem to struggle with this; once a thought has occurred to them, they have a lot more trouble dismissing it, as the parts of the brain that would normally help them dismiss it seem to be disrupted in some way.

An interesting link to addiction is that, with OCD and similar, there is evidence that points to a problem in the opiate system of the brain. On a more day-to-day level, some argue that the opiate system and the endorphins it runs on are involved in the processes that let us recognise when a task is done. We realise we need to lock our front door as we leave, we lock our front door, our opiate system fires up slightly, and this lets us know the job is done and we can move on. It allows us to dismiss things and move on. But in those with OCD, it's suggested that this opiate system activity doesn't occur, or is insufficient, for some reason. And so, they end up repeating the same thought or action, long after it's necessary.[17] As ever, there's a lot going on in the brain here.

Just to make it one hundred per cent clear: I'm not saying addiction doesn't involve impulse control problems, or compulsions. Because of course it does. And those with impulse control issues or compulsive disorders tend to be at a higher risk of becoming addicts. But it's important to recognise that you can have these issues *without* addiction, so they shouldn't all be lumped together.

It's a tricky one, though, making reliable distinctions between all these things. Interestingly, the DSM and the ICD take different approaches here. The latest edition of the DSM included gambling addiction in the addictive disorders category. But nothing else made the cut. Not sex addiction, not kleptomania, not shopping addiction, not smartphone addiction. As far as the DSM is concerned, these things aren't addictions. Not that the DSM dismisses them outright – they're included, sometimes as impulse disorders, or compulsions, but often in appendices, or similar. In essence, the DSM is saying, 'Not sure about these ones, we need more data.'

However, the latest volume of the ICD deviates from the DSM approach, and does include gaming disorder as an addictive condition. So, according to the World Health Organization, who produce the ICD, you *can* be addicted to video games.* Similarly, the latest ICD includes pyromania, kleptomania, pathological gambling, compulsive sexual disorder, and more, as confirmed mental health issues. Admittedly, they're classed as impulse control disorders, not addictions, but who knows what the next volume will bring?

This isn't consistent with what the DSM says. Why? Well, the DSM is written by, and typically *for*, psychiatrists, primarily in the US and developed countries. So, the specifics are very important, because they're often used to determine treatment options. The ICD, by contrast, is a global publication from the World Health Organization, so is more a tool for deciding who needs help and why, often in poorer countries with minimal mental health infrastructure. The purpose of the ICD is to make it easier for those who need help to

---

* It seems my mother was right all along.

get it. By including more possible diagnoses, disorders are more likely to be logged or picked up, so those that need it are more likely to get the intervention and assistance they require. So, it's perhaps unsurprising that the criteria and parameters for diagnoses sometimes deviate from the DSM, which is primarily about making sure people get the correct help they need, when help is available.

The fact that diagnoses can differ and fluctuate so much brings us back to the original issues raised in the first chapter, which pointed out how the very concept of diagnoses can be limited and problematic. In any case, assuming we can be sure that someone has an addiction, what can be done about it?

The treatment of addicts

Drug addiction is undoubtedly the most common form of addiction, so most treatments focus on that. Rehab is a very commonplace term. It pops up often in the mainstream, usually in the context of high-profile celebrities with drug problems who need to sober up. Rehab is, as you probably knew already, short for rehabilitation, as in rehabilitation clinics. Big-name celebs and wealthy types are often seen checking in to particularly luxurious ones, in exotic locations amid sun-kissed beaches, and catered by gourmet chefs. Because when you're obscenely rich, why shouldn't your cold turkey be exquisitely prepared? Although, if you're guaranteed to be experiencing severe discomfort from withdrawal, it probably helps to have all the other aspects of your environment be as pleasant as possible.

That's a particularly expensive version, sure, but all rehab clinics follow the same basic model: a secure environment, where someone can detox in safety. Round-the-clock medical observation in safe, but tightly regulated, environments means a patient can get the drug out of their system with minimal risk to themselves. They get the assistance they need, but no opportunity to obtain the source of their addiction, so it's not just a matter of willpower.

Rehab clinics often include therapy sessions, as these are another common approach for dealing with addiction. CBT or group therapies can be very useful to help uncover and deal with issues that led to addictions to begin with, or to instil a sense of self-worth and social bonding in those who lack such things, which is bleakly common after long bouts of addiction. It might sound wishy-washy, but it's often a crucial part of recovery, because if you're convinced that nobody gives a damn about you, including yourself, why *bother* to fight an addiction? Talking therapies – psychotherapeutic interventions – are many and varied, because exactly what leads someone to addiction, and why, is often very specific to that person. Getting to the bottom of the causes and issues, and resolving them, can be a drawn-out but pivotal process.

It's not entirely down to the addict to do the legwork themselves, thankfully. There are medications available for addiction. We've looked at methadone, but there are also things like buprenorphine and naltrexone, which help manage the worst symptoms of withdrawal and dependence, including reducing nausea and pain sensitivity. Both are big problems, particularly in opiate withdrawal.

286

There are also more 'tough love' interventions, which effectively force an addict to abstain. Disulfiram (trade name Antabuse) is a drug that makes someone extremely sensitive to alcohol, meaning alcohol makes them physically ill. It blocks the breakdown of alcohol in the body, so alcohol consumption causes an extreme hangover immediately, with all the headaches, vomiting, and more. Even in small doses. And when I say small, I mean it. Taking Antabuse means you need to avoid anyone wearing an alcohol-based aftershave or scent, because even that can cause a reaction.

There is also the usual range of psychoactive medications, such as antidepressants, antipsychotics and anxiolytics, because if the addiction does stem from a desperate attempt to relieve a pre-existing mental health problem, getting that issue under control will be a big help. These drugs also help control the more specific aspects of an addiction, such as the impulse control problems, the compulsions, the withdrawal, and more.

All these interventions, from the crude to the nuanced, are generally meant to help an addict break the cycle of addiction, enabling them to abstain from their drug, or behaviour, for long enough that their brains and bodies can revert to a more sustainable state – one that isn't reliant on the drug. Although, as stated, the changes brought about by addiction often don't go away entirely. Hence why relapse can be so common, and many a recovering addict is constantly vigilant, and must swear off their addiction entirely. They can't just dabble, have a cheeky drink or puff here or there. They play the long game, because their brains are still primed to go back to the old ways. All the systems of addiction are technically still in there, they're just powered down, so to speak.

Remember the analogy of the town where the stadium appears? And how much chaos it causes? Well, even if the town manages to return to some semblance of normal when the stadium vanishes, a lot of the changes and developments, like the new buildings and altered roads, and all the people who liked having the lucrative stadium crowds around, will still be there. If the stadium were to suddenly reappear, these things would quickly go right back to work, and you'd end up in the same intense, unsustainable situation you'd worked so hard to get away from. You couldn't just have the stadium appear every now and again, as and when you felt like it. Once it's gone, it needs to *stay* gone. And this is true for most addicts – once the drug is out of their life, it needs to *stay* out.

This, though, is the *end* result of many addictions. It's worth noting that one of the main focuses of treatment of addiction is at the very beginning, getting the individual to accept that there's a problem to be dealt with at all. And we've seen why this is often a struggle. Accordingly, psychologists have come up with the transtheoretical, or 'states of change', model of addiction.[18] It describes the addict as being in one of five possible stages: pre-contemplation, contemplation, decision, action and maintenance.

In the pre-contemplation stage, the addict doesn't know, or at least doesn't accept or admit, that they have an issue. Contemplation is when they do acknowledge it and contemplate doing something about it. Decision is when they take the plunge and decide to address their issue. Action is, predictably, where they actually do something about it, and maintenance is, as you'd assume, maintaining their new, recovered situation by avoiding triggers or things linked to their addiction. A failing or loss of motivation during any of the latter two stages can lead to relapse, a sadly rather common occurrence.

There is also some concern with the labelling of addiction as a disease, or illness. A lot of people push the idea that addiction is definitely an illness or disease, and for good reason, given how hard it is already for addiction to be acknowledged as a problem deserving of care and help. But, while well meant, it harks back to earlier, where we saw the downsides of treating mental health problems as standard medical disorders. Specifically, the aspect where the patient is expected to remain largely passive in the process. This is regularly an unhelpful approach to mental health problems anyway, but it's particularly true with addiction, where the motivation and commitment of the patient is often the deciding factor for recovery.

That's one argument anyway. Other people disagree. There are many problems thrown up when dealing with addiction. Even the word addiction has a chequered history.

Dependence or addiction, addiction or dependence?

Some of you reading this may have been surprised, even annoyed, by the fact that, throughout this chapter, I've constantly used the terms addicts and addiction. You might want to point out to me that people aren't defined by their disorders, and addiction is not the technical term for such a complex issue. Someone who spent so long explaining the importance of accuracy and care in the language used to describe mental health should surely not be so blasé, so cavalier, when deploying terms like addict. All good points. But I promise there hasn't been some clumsy lapse on my part. My use of the terms addict and addiction was deliberate. And here's why.

In the previous version of the DSM, the DSM-4, the words addiction, addict or addictive weren't used. No, the label was substance abuse and dependence disorders. Apparently, this was the subject of much debate, with the mental health community being split on whether the term addiction should be used.[19] The term dependence eventually won out by the narrowest of margins, because it was feared that the term addiction is so freighted with stigma and judgement that potential patients would be put off from seeking help they genuinely need, thus making the situation a lot worse. A more neutral term like drug dependence doesn't have as much weight or negativity attached to it.

However, this led to a problem, because the term dependence was already in use. Dependence is a part of addiction, sure, hence withdrawal happens when the source of the addiction is removed. Because the individual *depends* on it. But you can be dependent on something, usually a drug, *without* being addicted to it. Many long-term users of antidepressants are dependent on them, as they experience withdrawal symptoms if they give them up too quickly, or at all. But they often aren't addicted to them; taking them isn't pleasurable, and they'd happily give them up if that didn't invariably make things worse. Or, diabetics are undoubtedly dependent on insulin, but are they addicted to it? A diabetic denied insulin would presumably go to great lengths to get it back, but this would be completely logical behaviour.

In fairness, earlier in this chapter I did say that long-term addicts are in a similar situation – they need to take their drug just to stave off withdrawal and all the awful consequences of that. There's no pleasure or enjoyment involved any more. They could definitely be said to be dependent on their drug to function, as many addicts are.

But the difference is, this is only the final, later stages of an addiction. And it's not *just* that, in addiction. There's everything else too: the denial, the distorted thinking, the compulsions, the poor impulse control, the preoccupation with the drug, the habits and cravings, all that. You rarely get any of that with people dependent on antidepressants, or insulin. You usually just get the sometimes reluctant acceptance that they need their particular substance in order to function. And that's where the confusion starts. Being dependent on a drug is a part of addiction, but not the whole story. And you can be dependent without being addicted. Using dependence as an all-encompassing label omits this aspect.

However, in the latest volume, the DSM has opted to bring back the term addiction, and variations thereof. It's partly because teaching medics and other students about drug dependence was tricky, when the term was used for both a biological dependence and substance abuse or related issues. A lot of confusion occurred, and when you're teaching medicine and healthcare, that can be very bad. There's also the fact that avoiding it meant the label 'addiction' retained its negative connotations, as it was used mostly by those who are less informed, or have a dubious ideological agenda to push.

But the main reason the dependence label was dropped in favour of addiction was that clinicians and doctors were regularly under-prescribing painkillers to those who needed them. Basically, you've got a generation of medics who've been taught that dependence is the same as addiction. So, if someone keeps asking for pain medication, they're clearly dependent on it, so are addicted, or close to, and should be cut off, lest you make the problem worse. This is wrong, though. Genuine addiction resulting from pain relief is surprisingly rare. Why would this be?

Well, remember, a big part of addiction involves overstimulation of the reward pathway. If you introduce powerful painkillers into a normal brain, it seriously ramps up the reward pathway via artificial means, causing all the unhelpful outcomes we've covered in depth. But what if you introduce powerful painkillers into a brain that's experiencing serious pain? That's not an excess of pleasure, that's a removal of pain and discomfort. Pain is, at the most basic level, a signal for your body and brain that something is *wrong,* and drugs like opiates can remove it. This might not seem like much, but it's a key difference, one the brain recognises, because it's a very smart organ.

Essentially, introducing drugs like opiates into a normal brain causes an intense pleasure response, which is unusual. It's beyond the normal functioning of the brain, and the brain recognises this, so responds to deal with it, bringing about all the changes we've discussed that typically lead to addiction.

But a brain that's experiencing severe pain? Introduce opiates here and the pain is removed. So, the drugs don't push the brain beyond its normal limits; they *remove a problem*, they restore normal functioning to the brain. That's arguably the key difference. If drugs disrupt normal processes, the brain adapts, changes, to deal with them, leading to addiction. If drugs cause the brain to return to, or remain in, normal parameters, the brain doesn't need to adapt, so addiction is far less likely. Presumably the same applies to antidepressants and insulin; there's no extreme pleasure response, there's just a maintenance of normal functioning. Ergo, nothing to get addicted to.

So, back to the original point, about doctors denying people painkillers for fear of causing an addiction. This was a bad policy, because those asking for painkillers are usually doing so because they're in serious pain! They are genuinely dependent on painkillers to function. But clinicians were less willing to prescribe them for fear of creating an addiction, because they've been taught that dependence is the same as addiction. Even though it isn't.

And so, the addiction label was reinstated to describe someone with the relevant disorder. It may seem like splitting hairs, but this is a stark example of what I was getting at in the very first chapter. Namely, when it comes to mental health, words matter! Using the wrong word to describe addiction genuinely led to countless people suffering needlessly. That's why I've been using the terms addiction and addict wherever possible. These should be neutral terms. Perhaps if I say them often enough, they will be?

However, I'm not that hopelessly optimistic. The sad thing is, the judgement and stigma linked to addiction aren't straightforward. They're tightly bound up with many of the inequalities of the modern world.

Addicted to harmful stigma

As well as reintroducing the term addiction, the new DSM also dropped a criterion from the addictive disorders category. It was 'committing illegal acts'. So, from now on, your tendency to break the law, or not, won't affect whether you get an addiction diagnosis. Does this make sense?

Granted, the cognitive changes brought about by addiction can, and often do, make someone prioritise obtaining their drug over obeying the law. But is that medically relevant? Clearly, experts now say no. So, they dropped it.

Like diagnosis itself, the law isn't consistent. Laws change, they come and go. Take someone who enjoys cannabis. And let's say they warrant a diagnosis of mild addictive disorder, as they meet just two criteria. They smoke way more than they'd like. And they're committing illegal acts, because they're regularly buying cannabis, the source of their addiction, which is against the law. But then, a week later, cannabis is legalised in their country. Now they *don't* meet the criteria for an addictive disorder, as they're not doing anything illegal. Last week they warranted a medical diagnosis, this week they don't. But they're not doing anything different. They've not changed at all.

Basing a diagnosis on something as variable as the laws of the land can be tantamount to mooring your boat by tying it to a cow. It's a big, heavy, solid thing, sure, but you can't guarantee it's not going to wander off and take you with it.

But on a more social level, including 'committing illegal acts' in the actual diagnostic criterion fundamentally links addiction to criminality. And if anything's going to perpetuate the already serious stigma, it's that. Because while addiction will never *not* be a serious issue, it is made substantially more serious by the judgement, condemnation and punishment heaped upon addicts. And this punishment isn't doled out logically or fairly. Much of it is down to prejudice and privilege.

Addiction is tightly bound up with drugs, obviously. And drugs are illegal and widely vilified in many countries and societies (even if they've been an integral part of most of them for centuries). The general view is that drugs are bad, and if you use them, you're a bad, flawed or inferior person. Harsh prison sentences are often meted out to those found guilty of selling or even possessing illegal drugs, by way of deterrent.

However, how bad and wrong drugs are, and how awful you are for using them, varies widely depending on your social standing.

A young man from an impoverished background, who grew up in a high-crime area, who is regularly smoking

crack cocaine in a dirty squat? He's bad, dirty, wrong, criminal, lock him up! But a very similar guy, same age, same
height, same appearance, earning half a million a year in a
prominent media job because he went to all the right schools
and his dad owns the company, constantly snorting cocaine
off the toilet seats in the tastefully decorated bathrooms of
exclusive nightclubs? He's a high-flyer, up-and-comer, party
animal, living life to the fullest. Perks of the job. And so on.

Let's say both these guys are addicted to drugs. In fact,
the rich guy is getting through twice as much cocaine as
the poor guy. But will he face as much stigma? Judgement?
Prejudice? Punishment? Not even close. Consider the number of people who've talked openly about rampant cocaine
use in the media and business worlds, particularly in the
eighties. It's featured prominently in countless films and TV
shows. Technically, every single user is a criminal. Are they
ever portrayed as such? Rarely.

And contrast the number of impoverished people who
face harsh fines and life-ruining prison sentences if they're
caught with drugs at a young age with all the wealthy polit-
icians who brag about their youthful drug experimentation.*
Why do they get a pass? Do they have brains with different properties that render them immune to addiction? No,
there's no such thing. We just don't seem to equate addiction

---

* In the 2019 Conservative Party leadership contest, many of the candidates were revealed to have dabbled in drugs, sometimes even class-A
ones. None were penalised for it, even though they were competing for
the role of *actual leader of the United Kingdom*! But they had all gone to
Oxford or similarly prestigious universities, so it was fine. Apparently.

with those in positions of power, even though they can often be more prone to it.

Indeed, the extent to which drug use is considered problematic is usually very context-dependent. It's often been said that what an American person would think of as dangerous alcohol consumption is what a British person would think of as an average night out. And it's only relatively recently that smoking has been deemed a bad thing to do, because in recent decades we had adverts everywhere encouraging it, and few people at the time saw a problem with that.

Is the same thing happening now? Think about how these days you can get shirts and posters and memes celebrating a reliance on caffeine. What if it's discovered in the next few years that it causes Alzheimer's? Are we still going to be so cavalier about our coffee enthusiasm? My point is, what counts as dangerous drug use is a slippery concept, as much as anything else, and can vary considerably from place to place and time to time, let alone person to person. And those on the receiving end of judgement and stigma are invariably those on the lowest rungs of the societal ladder, the impoverished and already maligned.

Given the scope of addiction we've covered and how it works, wealth and privilege should be no defence against it. And they aren't. But so many seem to blithely assume otherwise. And that doesn't help anybody, because it means the poorer addicts get punished more, while the wealthy ones are largely ignored, so can't or won't get any help for their issues. Is it any wonder so many famous people succumb to drug use and addiction? We seem to celebrate it in the higher-ups and condemn it harshly in those lower down. But the matter of who does and doesn't become addicted to something isn't determined by social standing.

No, there are other issues at work.

Who gets addicted? And why?

A big part of the stigma directed at addicts is the matter of choice. Nobody wants depression or anxiety or psychosis or PTSD, but it's not something they get to decide. But anyone with an addiction, they must have chosen to indulge in their vice at some point, right? Even if it was illegal? Therefore, addicts deserve less sympathy and more condemnation because their issues are self-inflicted.

But here's the thing: countless people try drugs, day in, day out. The majority do not become addicted. And I'd argue that no addict ever *planned* to become addicted, any more than a downhill skier plans to have broken legs. In truth, there's a great deal of evidence that shows that some people are simply more vulnerable to addiction. Certain genes, certain flukes of development, certain deficiencies or surpluses of chemicals, or other differences in how their brains work, mean that they have more difficulty with restraint or impulse control, or a drug hits them harder, or lasts longer, or whatever.

An interesting study from 2012 looked at fifty pairs of siblings, where in each pair one was addicted to cocaine and the other had no history of drug use.[20] Scanning the brains of their subjects, they regularly saw activity patterns that are strongly suggestive of impulse control deficits. They found

298

these in many of the cocaine users, as you'd probably expect. But more intriguingly, they also regularly found signs of the same impulse control deficits in the brains of the non-addicted siblings of the cocaine users. These siblings weren't drug users, but it implies they'd be more vulnerable to addiction if they ever decided to try them. These data strongly suggest there is some common factor hampering the impulse control processes in the related brains. Could it be some genetic trait they share? Or a common factor in the environment that they both grew up in? It could be either of these. Or something else.

This isn't to say poor impulse control is the sole cause of addiction. but it's undoubtedly something that increases the odds of developing an addiction, and this study, along with many others, reveals poor impulse control isn't just a lack of willpower, but something more fundamental in the make-up of an individual's brain.

Overall, there are many traits, genetic factors and internal properties a person can have, none of which they've any control over, which make them far more likely to develop an addiction. And this makes attributing blame and responsibility even more confusing. For instance, research shows that the aforementioned downhill skiers, the extreme ones who take increasingly mind-boggling risks, often have the thrill-seeking personality type. There's evidence linking this to genetic factors that mean they have reduced levels of receptors in their reward pathway.[21] One possible outcome of this is that they need more stimulation to achieve desired levels of pleasure, so engage in extreme risks.

Can they help their genetic make-up? No, they can't. If they end up severely injured, are they at fault? That's a murkier subject.

Addiction does seem to have a strong heritability to it. Many addicts saw their own parents struggle with addiction and swore never to let such a thing happen to them, but still ended up addicted, often to the same things that blighted their parents' lives.

Here's a story about exactly this from a Twitter friend, who requested to remain anonymous:

My father was a 'functioning alcoholic', and consumed large amounts of alcohol until it was an imminent mortal threat. I'm convinced it destroyed his marriage to my mother. As a teenager, I tried to convince him to quit many times, but that always went completely sideways. I vowed then to never drink. I witnessed the destruction it caused to his life, and I've lived with the damage it's done to my life. Yet, I got addicted to alcohol.

My mother died at fifty-nine of lung cancer, from a lifetime of smoking cigarettes. I had tried to get her to quit many times as well. She reacted far better than my father, bless her, but the outcome was the same. When she died, I had been smoking for fifteen years, and smoked for fifteen years after. And yes, when younger, I'd sworn I would never smoke.

People hearing this may think, 'Wow, you must be an extremely weak person.' But the fact that it did happen should prompt them to consider how intractable addiction

actually is. I maintained addictions to the very substances
that destroyed both of my parents, subsequently damaged a
huge portion of my life, and likely will shorten it as well.

I'm not being hyperbolic when I say addiction is a
monster of Godzilla proportions. Lay-folk who have not
suffered it have no idea at all how horrific it is inside the
addict's mind. None.

The genetic element is important, but we must also remember
that the human brain is extremely adept at learning from our
environment, and particularly from those around us, regarding what's right or wrong, good or bad. Especially when compared to abstract facts and information. There's a vast body of
information out there about how the universe and physics and
nature all work. And yet, people born and raised in devoutly
religious households almost invariably believe the teachings of
that religion, no matter how incompatible with the evidence
they may be.

Because what we learn from others, from those with whom
we associate, often carries far more weight than abstract data,
than intangible facts and claims, no matter how legitimate
they may be. And because we want to fit in, to belong, the
behaviours and views of others are more influential again.
Therefore, someone who grows up in an environment or community where drug-taking is treated as normal, or at least
nothing to panic about, is far more likely to internalise these
messages and not recognise the risks of taking them.

You could argue that it's no excuse, that everyone knows
drugs are bad, and illegal, and that anyone who ignores

these warnings deserves all they get. But then, we all know speeding is illegal. Streaming TV shows and films and music without paying is illegal. Downloading free books from pirate sites is illegal. These things are all examples of breaking the law, but countless people do them anyway, and argue that it's fine because 'everyone does it'.

See what I'm getting at? The threat of the law rarely wins when it's up against the community consensus. So, if everyone around you takes drugs, the fact that they're illegal wouldn't carry much weight. And this is all assuming you have no pre-existing issues that would predispose you to addiction. For many addicts, that's not the case. There are all those inherited factors I mentioned. What if you already have an impulse control disorder? Or a compulsion? Both often lead you to do things you know aren't wise while limiting your ability to stop yourself. People with these issues regularly develop addictions, as the odds are stacked against them already.

And as I stated way back at the start of this chapter, close to half of people with mental health problems already end up involved with substance abuse, or similar. Because, far too often, there's precious little alternative available for them when it comes to getting even minor relief from their issues. What chance have they got?

Addiction: mental health in miniature

The reason I wanted to talk about addiction in such depth was because, in my humble opinion, it represents the current state of mental health in general. People with addiction have long been stigmatised, scorned, mocked, judged and persecuted. Although that situation has improved in recent years, there is still a very long way to go in undoing these preconceptions.

The same goes for those with mental health problems in general.

For the longest time, it was assumed that addiction was due to some personal, moral or even ethical failing. Scientific developments have shown that this is by no means the case, and a lot of it is down to issues and changes in the brain that the individual has no control over.

The same goes for those with mental health problems in general.

The terminology used when discussing addiction can have surprisingly broad, and potent, consequences for those dealing with it.

The same goes for those with mental health problems in general.

For much of recent history, addiction has been thought of and spoken about almost exclusively in terms of chemicals, and how they affect our brains. But recent developments have shown that behaviours and environments and contexts are a far more significant factor than previously assumed.

The same goes for those with mental health problems in general.

You could say that addiction is the result of the more sophisticated parts of the human brain, and the world these have allowed us to create, pushing the simpler fundamental regions beyond their limits, causing confusion and disruption.

The same goes for those with mental health problems in general.

Our understanding and perception of addiction is far more dependent on cultural norms, prejudices and subjective assumptions than most people would ever assume. As a result, it's constantly in flux, and subject to change all the time.

The same goes for those with mental health problems in general.

There are still those who insist that addiction *isn't* a mental disorder. But based on all this, I can't see how you could think it's anything else.

I point this out because if you're someone who champions mental health problems but condemns addicts as inferior, you're not really helping.

6: Conclusion

At this point, you've read about 80,000 words about mental health, and will have dedicated several hours of your life to doing so. Despite this, I've barely scratched the surface of mental health. Actually, even that's an optimistic analysis. At best, I've successfully pointed in the general direction of the surface of mental health.

There's just so much about it to consider, and it affects literally every level of our beings. Many of the finest minds in the world are working round the clock to figure it out, and they're still a long way off. No way am I going to be able to deal with it comprehensively in one single book. Sure, I won't deny that I've managed to go into some exhaustive detail: about how mental health is perceived and dealt with overall, about the workings of the brain, about depression, about anxiety, and about addiction. But I'm fully aware that there's a lot more that I *didn't* get around to covering.

There are many other classes and types of mental health problems. Psychotic disorders, like schizophrenia, are familiar to many people, and there's a whole world of stigma and misconceptions to be tackled there. Same goes for personality disorders. Eating disorders have their own particular properties and effects, as well as being something almost uniquely human and modern. There's a lot they could tell us, if we were to investigate them.

I mentioned obsessive compulsive disorder briefly, but

305

didn't go into nearly as much detail as I'd like. Same goes for mania, and bipolar disorders. In fact, there are multiple issues and problems that I mentioned in passing that definitely deserve full chapters of their own.

Then there are the other disorders that many people often mistakenly categorise as mental health problems, despite actually being different things, and this difference can tell us a lot. These include neurological disorders, like Alzheimer's and Parkinson's, and neurodevelopmental disorders, like ADHD and autism. They're considered distinct from mental health issues, as the underlying mechanism is more physical in nature, such as certain parts of the brain starting to degrade and die off; or there's an issue or problem that occurs in the development of the brain, which has, predictably, lasting consequences for how said brain works and operates.

Undeniably, such disorders, of the neurological or neuro-developmental sort, can, and regularly do, impact on an individual's mental health, so you see a lot of mental health problems in people with these conditions. But, in many ways, the mental health aspects are more downstream from the main problem, not the problem in and of itself. So, they're classed differently. Does that make sense?*

So, there are many different forms of mental health problems out there that I've not even mentioned. I've focused on depression, anxiety and addiction largely because they're the most common, most familiar, most recognisable. There's no value judgement here; I'm not arguing that these disorders or

* I'm aware that much of this doesn't, at least on first reading.

CONCLUSION

issues are the best, worst, most important, or anything like that.
I've just gone with the numbers, largely so I can just blame the
abstract data if anyone wants to question me about it.

And I don't doubt that they will. I said it at the start, and
I'm going to say it again now: it's pretty much guaranteed
that anyone who reads this book will find something, if not
many things, that they disagree with. We've seen how subjective, how constantly in flux the general understanding of
mental health is. There are so many subjective and cultural
variations regarding how it's defined, labelled, treated and
perceived. And these things change regularly, too.

Homosexuality was once a confirmed mental illness. Now
same-sex marriage is increasingly common. Addiction was
once a taboo word, then they realised this taboo was doing
more harm than good, so now it's back in the textbooks.
Heck, mental *illness* was, for a while, something people were
desperately trying to convince the wider world was a real
thing. Now you have people arguing that they should stop
doing that, because defining mental health problems as illnesses has consequences of its own.

Overall, certainty in the area of mental health is in short
supply. Because, when all's said and done, we're dealing with
the human mind. And there's nothing harder to pin down
than that, even when it's working normally. Which, in this
context, it isn't. That's why I tried to focus, where possible, on
the involvement of the brain and all its workings.

Not that the brain isn't a complex, baffling mess of things
itself. I've been in the neuroscience field for nearly two
decades now, but if you were to ask me to list all the things

I know about the brain that are one hundred per cent established irrefutable facts, I'd run out of facts before I ran out of fingers to count them on. But at least the brain has a physical presence. We can look at it, we can poke it, we can interfere with it and see what happens.

And so, in this book, we've seen what seems to happen in a brain experiencing mental health problems. A lot of it seems to involve stress, particularly at the neurological level. Constant stress, over prolonged periods, is something our modern world is very generous with. It's also seemingly the Achilles heel of the long-established workings of the modern brain. Stress is a normal reaction to adverse occurrences, with countless complicated physical and chemical effects. But because the human brain is as flexible and adaptable as it is, making it experience these effects for long periods means it causes unhelpful changes, which affect how we think and function.

Stress can overstimulate the key regions of the brain linked to fear and apprehension, so we get anxiety. This overstimulation can lead to vital brain regions becoming exhausted, stuck, unable to change, and this seems to be a key factor in depression. And when you're dealing with the effects of prolonged stress, you're more likely to turn to things that offer relief, like drink or drugs, which increases the likelihood of addiction. And addiction, both directly and indirectly, leads to more stress. It quickly becomes very self-sustaining.

Well, that's one theory anyway. There are others out there. Maybe the inflammation theory of depression has it right?[1] That's another thing I didn't even get around to mentioning!

Maybe it *is* all down to an overexpression of cortisol?

Maybe there's a currently unknown agent that causes the neurosteroids that maintain the GABA system to fail, and everything that occurs in anxiety and depression follows on from that?

There are other possibilities in the literature that I've not brought up. And no doubt many more that I've never heard of. It's a very big field, and a very changeable, very uncertain one.

So, what was the point of all this? If I think I'm just spitting in the wind, why did I write this book in the first place?

Well, part of it was that I wanted to provide some clarity as to the ins and outs of mental health and associated practices, like psychiatry, psychology, psychotherapy, neurology, and more. There are so many different claims and viewpoints about how mental health does or should work, but so many of these are heavily influenced by personal experiences, beliefs, investments and ideologies. That's why they regularly get so heated, meaning discussions quickly get derailed.

I don't claim to know who's right and wrong in the many ongoing disputes, but it was my hope to provide a more logical take on the issue. A Psycho-Logical one.* So, hopefully, after reading what I've written, you at least have a better idea of the lie of the land. You would hopefully be better able to recognise where people are coming from, why they say what they say, regarding mental health.

My other aim in writing this was to inform. Raising awareness remains a vital goal, but while many focus on promoting the message that mental health problems are a serious matter,

---

* And there's the title again. Clever, isn't it?

I figured it might be helpful to try to show *why* they're so serious. Because they are.

Over the course of this book, we've seen multiple ways in which something going awry in the brain, or the mind, can have numerous effects on someone's health, both physical and mental. No doubt there are still people who will insist that mental health problems are no big deal, or nothing to be concerned about, but we can now say with certainty that these people are wrong.*

Part of the problem is that there is a lot of conflicting information about mental health problems, how they work, how effective treatments are, and so on. Hopefully, after reading this book, you can now appreciate that, while a lot of mental health remains unclear or uncertain, there are numerous ways in which problems can be dealt with, or at least managed. The drugs and other therapies available aren't guaranteed to be effective, but nor are they a waste of time. They're basically what we've got, and how well they work varies from person to person.

And while I'm tempted to say that this shows there's nothing to worry about when it comes to mental health problems, I would never be that condescending or dismissive. Because of course there are plenty of things to worry about. If you've got anxiety, constant worrying is the whole problem! It's never fun or easy to have your mental health go awry. If it were, it wouldn't be an issue. My aim is that now, if you've read what I've written, and end up dealing with

* I mean, they were already wrong. But now they're even more wrong.

mental health problems of your own, you'll at least have a better idea of exactly what's going on, why it's happening. Sometimes a bit of clarity can make all the difference.

But I can sit here and prattle on about the lofty goals I had in writing this all I want. The truth is, I can only talk about this objectively. If you're dealing with mental health issues of your own, you technically know more about it than me.

I'll just be happy if I've helped in some way.

Glossary

Action potential – An electrochemical impulse, a 'spark', that travels along the **cell membrane** of neurons – brain cells – and allows them to transmit information. The neurological equivalent of the dots and dashes that make up Morse code.

Amino acid – A type of organic molecule. They are the building blocks of **proteins**. **Glutamate** is an amino acid.

Amygdala – A small but incredibly important brain region, located deep within the **temporal lobe**. While the amygdala is an important hub for emotional processes and is involved in many fundamental emotional reactions, it's mostly linked to producing fear and anxiety responses, when presented with threat or danger.

Anterior cingulate cortex – A neurological region, located behind the very front of the brain. It's involved in important processes like attention and focus, impulse control, self-awareness, and more.

Basolateral nucleus – Also known as the basolateral **amygdala**, or basolateral complex. It's a specific part of the amygdala, into which sensory and other information from elsewhere in the brain is fed and the relevant emotional response is determined.

Cell – Microscopic self-contained chemical structures, cells are the fundamental building block of all Earth-based life. All living organisms, all their organs and tissues, are made of cells.

Cell membrane – The surrounding complex molecular layer, the 'skin', of a cell that holds it together and controls what can go into and out of a cell.

Cellular medium – The environment in which a cell exists and by which it is sustained. If it's inside a body, the medium is the **interstitial fluid**. If it's a cell in a Petri dish or similar, it's the fluid or buffer substance contained in the dish.

Chemical messenger – Any chemical that is released by one cell/tissue that can be detected by another. Upon detection of the chemical messenger, the recipient cell/tissue changes what it's doing. **Neurotransmitters** and **hormones** are the main forms of chemical messenger.

Cortex – The upper layer of the brain, the large wrinkled mass on top. In humans, the cortex is by far the biggest part of the brain. It contains all the regions associated with our most complex abilities (e.g. thinking, planning, self-awareness etc.) but still has many extensive links with the more fundamental regions and processes lower down in the brain. It is sometimes known as the 'neocortex'.

Corticotrophin-releasing factor – A **hormone** that plays an important role in our brain and body's physical response to stress. It's often found in abnormally high concentrations in blood samples of those enduring severe mental health problems or similarly stressful experiences.

Cortisol – The most famous 'stress **hormone**', released into the bloodstream at times of stress. It causes many of the known physiological effects of prolonged stress. **Corticotrophin-releasing factor** is a precursor chemical; its presence in certain tissues causes the release of cortisol.

Depressive episode – The period ranging from the onset of an individual experiencing the clinically recognised symptoms of depression, until they cease, and more normal mental functioning returns. The length of a depressive episode can vary considerably depending on the type of depression (or related disorder).

DNA – Deoxyribonucleic Acid. The famous double helix molecule found in nearly all **cells**. It provides a means of storing and sharing vast amounts of microscopic information, and thus acts as the effective blueprint for every part of our body.

DNA code – A way of referring to the information in our DNA that dictates our eventual physical properties, e.g. 'You have brown eyes because they're written into your DNA code.' Also known as 'Genetic Code'.

Dynorphin – A type of **neurotransmitter**, one widely believed to play many important roles in our experiences of pain and stress.

Frontal lobe – One of the four main lobes that make up the brain. Located at the very front of the brain. It is typically where our most complex cognitive processes occur; it contains the **prefrontal cortex**, an especially important collection of brain regions in this regard.

GABA (Gamma-AminoButyric Acid) – A **neurotransmitter**, the most well-known inhibitory kind. This means that the presence of GABA invariably leads to cellular processes being *suppressed*, not stimulated.

Gene – A particular sequence of **DNA** that encodes for something specific, usually a type of **protein** essential for

314

the structure of our bodies. If DNA were a block of text, genes would be the individual words found within it.

Glia – The **cells** that make up our nervous system, but which aren't **neurons**. They don't transmit signals; they instead provide structural support and maintenance for neurons, and are thus also a crucial element of the nervous system.

Glucocorticoid – A type of steroid **hormone**, another one that is typically released in response to stress. As well as physical effects like suppressing our immune response, it's also known to act on key areas of the brain that regulate our focus and memory when we're feeling stressed.

Glutamate – The most abundant neurotransmitter in the brain, with a very wide range of functions. Glutamate is an excitatory neurotransmitter; it stimulates (increases the activity of) the neurons it interacts with.

Hippocampus – A region of the **temporal lobe**, where new memories are created. The hippocampus is also involved in retrieving existing memories. It looks a bit like a seahorse (Latin: hippocampus), hence its name.

Hormone – A type of **chemical messenger**, alongside **neurotransmitters**. Hormones are released into the bloodstream and affect organs and tissues elsewhere in the body.

Hypothalamus – A neurological region located below the **thalamus**, it is effectively where the brain and body 'meet', where what goes on in the brain can directly affect the workings of the body, typically via release of **hormones** into the bloodstream.

Impulse control disorder – A condition whereby an individual has a reduced ability to consciously control or overrule subconscious impulses and tendencies, be they emotional, reflexive, habit-based, etc. These can manifest in a wide range of ways.

Insular cortex – A region located deep in the brain at the boundary between several lobes. It has important roles in multiple processes, including self-awareness, consciousness and motor control. It is also a key region in the brain's ability to experience disgust.

Interstitial fluid – Also known as 'extracellular fluid', it describes all the fluid in a body that isn't found inside cells. It typically provides the **cell medium**, so is vitally important.

Ion – Charged atoms. Typical atoms are made up of neutrons, protons and electrons. Protons have a positive electrical charge, while electrons have a negative one. They usually balance each other out, so the overall charge of the atom is zero. Ions are atoms with a positive or negative charge, due to possessing too few or too many electrons, respectively.

Limbic system – The collection of brain regions responsible for processing emotions. Although the idea of a centralised and anatomically distinct part of the brain that deals specifically with emotions is no longer considered realistic in light of more recent evidence that suggests emotions are processed by most parts of the brain, 'the limbic system' is still used as an umbrella term to describe the emotional processes in the brain.

Membrane potential – **Cell membranes** have different concentrations of ions either side of them, meaning the inside and outside of a cell has a different degree of electrical charge. This sets up a microscopic voltage, known as the membrane potential. *Resting* membrane potential describes the voltage that occurs when the cell isn't doing anything, beyond the basics needed to stay alive. It's like describing the amount of energy being used by a TV on standby.

Monoamine hypothesis – The theory that depression in humans is the result of reduced levels of certain **neurotransmitters** (i.e. monoamine neurotransmitters) in the brain, meaning neurological activity is impaired in many ways, which results in depression. More recent findings and enhanced understanding have shown the monoamine hypothesis to be, at best, an oversimplification of the reality, but it still has a lot of influence over our understanding of depression, particularly in the mainstream.

Monoamine oxidase inhibitor – An earlier class of antidepressants. They're still used today, usually when more recently developed antidepressant types have proven ineffective. Monoamine oxidase is a type of **protein** (known as an enzyme) that removes certain **neurotransmitters** from the brain, after they're used. Monoamine oxidase inhibitors prevent this happening, thus increasing the levels of the relevant neurotransmitters (see **monoamine hypothesis**).

Neuroendocrine – Referring to something that is involved in both the nervous system and the endocrine (i.e. **hormone**) system. The **hypothalamus** is the most obvious example; it's part of the brain (so part of the nervous system) that releases a lot of hormones into the blood-stream (so is part of the endocrine system).

Neurohormone – A chemical messenger that can act as both a **hormone** and a **neurotransmitter**, such as oxytocin or vasopressin. [Most of the hormones referred to in this book are technically neurohormones].

Neuron – The primary cells that make up the brain and nervous system, which are responsible for all that the brain does. Neurons can communicate and share information with each other, via **action potentials**, **neurotransmitters**, and more. They can be excitatory (i.e. cause more activity in a connecting neuron) or inhibitory (reduce or stop activity in a connection neuron). How the neurons in our brains are connected dictates much of who we are and what we're capable of.

Neuroplasticity – The ability of neurons to adapt and change in response to new stimulation and experiences. It was long believed that neurons in the mature adult brain lacked neuroplasticity (i.e. were 'fixed') but more recent evidence shows otherwise. Changes and deficiencies in neuroplasticity are believed to underpin numerous mental health problems.

Neurosteroid – An important class of chemical supplied to neurons by **glia**, to maintain neuron health and functionality.

Neurotransmitter – A type of chemical messenger. **Neurons** send neurotransmitters to each other to rapidly pass on signals and information. There are a wide range of types and classes of neurotransmitters, with differing roles and effects. Neurotransmitters are to **hormones** what emails are to physical letters.

Nucleus accumbens – A small region deep within the brain, it is mostly known for being one end of the **reward pathway**. It is responsible for providing the sensation of reward (i.e. pleasure) we experience when something good happens.

Occipital lobe – One of the four main lobes that make up the brain. The occipital lobe is found at the rear of the brain, and contains much of the visual processing areas.

Orbitofrontal cortex – A part of the **prefrontal cortex**, it's a region often linked to self-control, via roles in emotional evaluation and predictions of the outcomes of actions.

Parietal lobe – One of the four main lobes that make up the brain. It's located in the upper-middle region of the **cortex** and is made up of many varied areas, involving movement control, sensory processes, and more.

Periaqueductal grey – A small neurological region found low down in the midbrain, the forward-most part of the brainstem. It has many crucial roles, including detecting and responding to threats, and modulation of the pain response.

Prefrontal cortex – A cluster of regions in the **frontal cortex**, most of which are involved in, or responsible for, our most complex cognitive abilities. If our sense of identity, our 'self', dwells anywhere in the brain, it's likely to be the prefrontal cortex.

Protein – Large, complex and endlessly variable organic molecules. Made up of long chains of **amino acids**, they perform many vital roles in our bodies, such as providing

319

cell structure, sending messages, fighting infections, and more.

Psychoactive – A chemical (usually a drug) that changes your mental state by altering the workings or activity of the brain and nervous system. *Psychotropic* is another familiar term that means the same thing.

Receptor (cell) – A molecule, usually a large and complex **protein**, embedded in the **cell membrane**, which interacts with a specific **chemical messenger**, and initiates a response in the presence of said messenger. Receptors are what chemical messengers interact with, to do their job.

Reward pathway – The small region in the centre of our brain, made up of the **nucleus accumbens, ventral tegmental area**, and the links between them, that allows us to feel pleasure in response to positive experiences. Recent evidence also suggests the existence of an 'anti-reward pathway', which is more diffuse throughout the brain, but acts in response to the reward pathway, to keep it in check and discourage too much pleasure-seeking.

Serotonin system – The neurons and neural networks in our brains that use the **neurotransmitter** serotonin, the most common target of antidepressant drugs. It was previously believed that there was only one serotonin system spread throughout the brain, like an underground train network serving a city, but recent evidence suggests there are multiple serotonin systems that may work against each other, like a city with competing bus routes.

Stress hormone – Chemicals (e.g. **cortisol**) released into the bloodstream by various organs and tissues in response to a stressful event or experience. They typically produce all the known physical symptoms of stress (e.g. tension, impaired immune system etc.).

Stria terminalis – A region located centrally in the brain, which coordinates much of our response to stressful experiences.

Striatum – A moderately sized neurological region located in the centre of the brain. It incorporates many functions, meaning it is important for thinking, planning, decision-making and perception of reward. It has been the focus of much research as a result.

Substantia nigra – A region of the midbrain involved in reward processing and movement control. The substantia nigra can sometimes start to degenerate (i.e. the neurons it's made up of gradually die), and this is what causes Parkinson's disease.

Superior temporal gyrus – The part of the brain that includes, among other things, the auditory cortex, which allows us to hear, and speak and understand language.

Synapse – The 'gap' where two **neurons** meet. Neurons typically don't physically connect to each other, there's a space between them. This is the synapse. Neurons communicate across the synapse via **neurotransmitters**.

Temporal lobe – One of the four main lobes that make up the brain. The temporal lobe is located centrally and to the side. It contains the **hippocampus**, **amygdala** and many other crucial elements of the **limbic system**.

Thalamus – A vitally important 'hub' of the brain. Located near the centre, it acts as a relay and processing region for much of the information that's sent from one part of the brain to another. It has many crucial functions as a result.

Threat detection system – The elaborate network of neurological regions (including the **hippocampus**, **amygdala** and **periaqueductal grey**) that constantly monitors sensory information that may be interpreted as a threat or danger and triggers a fight-or-flight response (to varying degrees) if such a thing is detected. The threat detection system is a key part of stress and anxiety disorder.

Tricyclic amine – One of the earliest classes of antidepressants. Still in use today, but usually when more advanced classes of antidepressants prove ineffective.

Ventral tegmental area – One part of the **reward pathway**. It helps decide whether something warrants a pleasurable response.

References

Introduction

1 Greco, V. and Roger, D., 'Uncertainty, stress, and health', *Personality and Individual Differences*, 2003, 34(6): p. 1057–68.

1: The state of play

1 Boyd, K.M., 'Disease, illness, sickness, health, healing and wholeness: exploring some elusive concepts', *Medical Humanities*, 2000, 26(1): p. 9.

2 Sadeghfard, A., et al., 'The History of Melancholia Disease', *Iranian Journal of Medical Sciences*, 2016, 41(3 Suppl): p. S75.

3 Scholtz, M., 'Hippocrates' Aphorisms', *California and Western Medicine*, 1940, 52(3): p. 125–6.

4 Miserandino, C., 'The spoon theory', https://butyoudontlook sick.com, 2003.

5 Robinson, D.L., 'The IQ factor: implications for intelligence theory and measurement', *Personality and Individual Differences*, 1999, 27(4): p. 715–35.

6 Terrier, L.-M., Levêque, M., and Amelot, A., 'Most lobotomies were done on women', *Nature*, 2017, 548(7669): p. 523.

7 Simms, C. and Scowcroft, E., 'Suicide statistics report 2017', London, UK: Samaritans, December 2018.

8 Sharpe, M., et al., 'Integrated collaborative care for comorbid major depression in patients with cancer (SMaRT Oncology-2): a multicentre randomised controlled effectiveness trial', *The Lancet*, 2014, 384(9948): p. 1099–1108.

9   American Psychiatric Association, *Diagnostic and statistical manual of mental disorders (DSM-5*)*, APA Publishing (2013).

10 World Health Organization, *International Classification of Diseases, 11th Revision (ICD-11)*, 2018, www.who.int/classifications/icd/en/.

11 Sanacora, G., Treccani, G., and Popoli, M., 'Towards a glutamate hypothesis of depression: an emerging frontier of neuropsychopharmacology for mood disorders', *Neuropharmacology*, 2012, 62(1): p. 63–77.

12 Wakefield, J.C., 'DSM-5: An overview of changes and controversies', *Clinical Social Work Journal*, 2013, 41(2): p. 139–154.

13 Wakefield, J.C., 'DSM-5 grief scorecard: Assessment and outcomes of proposals to pathologize grief', *World Psychiatry*, 2013, 12(2): p. 171–3.

14 Stefan, M. and McManus, I., 'The concept of disease: its evolution in medical students', *Social Science and Medicine*, 1989, 29(7): p. 791–2.

15 Elkins, D.N., 'The medical model in psychotherapy: Its limitations and failures', *Journal of Humanistic Psychology*, 2009, 49(1): p. 66–84.

16 Kendler, K.S., 'The phenomenology of major depression and the representativeness and nature of DSM criteria', *American Journal of Psychiatry*, 2016, 173(8): p. 771–80.

17 Double, D., 'Giving up the disease model', *The Lancet Psychiatry*, 2015, 2(8): p. 682.

18 Beck, A.T. and Haigh, E.A., 'Advances in cognitive theory and therapy: The generic cognitive model', *Annual Review of Clinical Psychology*, 2014, 10: p. 1–24.

19 Yorke, C., 'Diagnosis in clinical practice: Its relationship to psychoanalytic theory', *The Psychoanalytic Study of the Child*, 1996, 51(1): p. 190–214.

20 Milton, J., 'Psychoanalysis and cognitive behaviour therapy – Rival paradigms or common ground?', *The International Journal of Psychoanalysis*, 2001, 82(3): p. 431–47.

21 Black, D.W., 'Efficacy of combined pharmacotherapy and psychotherapy versus monotherapy in the treatment of anxiety disorders', *CNS Spectrums*, 2006, 11(10 S12): p. 29–33.

22 Weitz, D., 'Struggling against psychiatry's human rights violations – an antipsychiatry perspective', *Radical Psychology*, 2008, 7: p. 7–8.

23 Garrett, M., '"Normalizing" the voice hearing experience: The continuum between auditory hallucinations and ordinary mental life' in Larøi, F. and Aleman, A. (Eds.), *Hallucinations: A guide to treatment and management* (Oxford University Press, 2010), p. 183–204.

24 Borrell-Carrió, F., Suchman, A.L., and Epstein, R.M., 'The biopsychosocial model 25 years later: principles, practice, and scientific inquiry', *The Annals of Family Medicine*, 2004, 2(6): p. 576–82.

2: How the brain works

1 Kasibhatla, R.D. and Russon, K., 'Femoral nerve blocks', *Journal of Perioperative Practice*, 2009, 19(2): p. 65–9.

2 Waggoner, A., 'Optical probes of membrane potential', *The Journal of Membrane Biology*, 1976, 27(1): p. 317–34.

3 Bean, B.P., 'The action potential in mammalian central neurons', *Nature Reviews Neuroscience*, 2007, 8(6): p. 451–65.

4 The Brainstorm Consortium, 'Analysis of shared heritability in common disorders of the brain', *Science*, 2018, 360(6395).

5 Nørremølle, A., et al., 'Trinucleotide repeat elongation in the Huntingtin gene in Huntington disease patients from 71

Danish families', *Human Molecular Genetics*, 1993, 2(9): p. 1475–6.

6   Fearnley, J.M. and Lees, A.J., 'Ageing and Parkinson's disease: substantia nigra regional selectivity', *Brain*, 1991, 114(5): p. 2283–301.

3: Depression

1   Lim, G.Y., et al., 'Prevalence of Depression in the Community from 30 Countries between 1994 and 2014', *Scientific Reports*, 2018, 8(1): p. 2861.

2   Vos, T., et al., 'Global, regional, and national incidence, prevalence, and years lived with disability for 301 acute and chronic diseases and injuries in 188 countries, 1990–2013: a systematic analysis for the Global Burden of Disease Study 2013', *The Lancet*, 2015, 386(9995): p. 743–800.

3   Hirschfeld, R., 'Bipolar spectrum disorder: improving its recognition and diagnosis', *The Journal of Clinical Psychiatry*, 2001, 62 (Suppl 14): p. 5–9.

4   Tsuno, N., Besset, A., and Ritchie, K., 'Sleep and depression', *The Journal of Clinical Psychiatry*, 2005, 66(10): p. 1254–69.

5   Segre, L.S., et al., 'The prevalence of postpartum depression', *Social Psychiatry and Psychiatric Epidemiology*, 2007, 42(4): p. 316–21.

6   Kelwala, S., Stanley, M., and Gershon, S., 'History of antidepressants: successes and failures', *The Journal of Clinical Psychiatry*, 1983, 44(5 Pt 2): p.40–8.

7   Hindmarch, I., 'Expanding the horizons of depression: beyond the monoamine hypothesis', *Human Psychopharmacology: Clinical and Experimental*, 2001, 16(3): p. 203–18.

8 Cipriani, A., et al., 'Comparative efficacy and acceptability of 21 antidepressant drugs for the acute treatment of adults with major depressive disorder: A systematic review and network meta-analysis', *The Lancet*, 2018, 391: p. 1357–66.

9 Ren, J., et al., 'Anatomically defined and functionally distinct dorsal raphe serotonin sub-systems', *Cell*, 2018, 175(2): p. 472–87. e20.

10 Krystal, J., et al., 'Glutamate and GABA systems as targets for novel antidepressant and mood-stabilizing treatments', *Molecular Psychiatry*, 2002, 7(1): p. S71–S80.

11 Liu, B., et al., 'From serotonin to neuroplasticity: Evolvement of theories for major depressive disorder', *Frontiers in Cellular Neuroscience*, 2017, 11: p. 305.

12 Burt, D.B., Zembar, M.J., and Niederehe, G., 'Depression and memory impairment: a meta-analysis of the association, its pattern, and specificity', *Psychological Bulletin*, 1995, 117(2): p. 285–305.

13 Meldrum, B.S., 'Glutamate as a neurotransmitter in the brain: review of physiology and pathology', *The Journal of Nutrition*, 2000, 130(4): p. 1007S–1015S.

14 Hashimoto, K., 'Rapid-acting antidepressant ketamine, its metabolites and other candidates: A historical overview and future perspective', *Psychiatry and Clinical Neurosciences*, 2019, 73(10): p. 613–27.

15 Palhano-Fontes, F., et al., 'A randomized placebo-controlled trial on the antidepressant effects of the psychedelic ayahuasca in treatment-resistant depression', bioRxiv, 2017: p. 103531.

16 Canady, V.A., 'FDA panel endorses ketamine nasal spray for depression', *Mental Health Weekly*, 2019, 29(8): p. 6–7.

327

17 Drobisz, D. and Damborská, A., 'Deep brain stimulation targets for treating depression', *Behavioural Brain Research*, 2019, 359: p. 266–73.

18 Heijnen, W.T.C., et al., 'Influence of age on ECT efficacy in depression and the mediating role of psychomotor retardation and psychotic features', *Journal of Psychiatric Research*, 2019, 109: p. 41–7.

19 Spinella, M., 'The role of prefrontal systems in sexual behavior', *International Journal of Neuroscience*, 2007, 117(3): p. 369–85.

20 Pittenger, C. and Duman, R.S., 'Stress, depression, and neuroplasticity: a convergence of mechanisms', *Neuropsychopharmacology*, 2008, 33(1): p. 88–109.

21 Pariante, C.M. and Lightman, S.L., 'The HPA axis in major depression: classical theories and new developments', *Trends in Neurosciences*, 2008, 31(9): p. 464–8.

22 Varghese, F.P. and Brown, E.S., 'The Hypothalamic-Pituitary-Adrenal Axis in Major Depressive Disorder: A Brief Primer for Primary Care Physicians', *Primary Care Companion to The Journal of Clinical Psychiatry*, 2001, 3(4): p. 151–5.

23 Rothstein, J.D., 'Excitotoxicity hypothesis', *Neurology*, 1996, 47(4 Suppl 2): p. 19S–26S.

24 Allen, N.B. and Badcock, P.B.T., 'Darwinian models of depression: A review of evolutionary accounts of mood and mood disorders', *Progress in Neuro-Psychopharmacology and Biological Psychiatry*, 2006, 30(5): p. 815–26.

4: Anxiety

1 Roese, N.J., 'Counterfactual thinking', *Psychological Bulletin*, 1997, 121(1): p. 133–148.

2   Mental Health Foundation, 'Statistics', published 2018;
    Available from: www.mentalhealth.org.uk/statistics.

3   Larson, C.L., et al., 'Recognizing threat: a simple geometric
    shape activates neural circuitry for threat detection', *Journal of
    Cognitive Neuroscience*, 2009, 21(8): p. 1523–35.

4   Teigen, K.H., 'Yerkes-Dodson: A law for all seasons', *Theory &
    Psychology*, 1994, 4(4): p. 525–47.

5   LeDoux, J., 'The amygdala', *Current Biology*, 2007, 17(20):
    p. R868–R874.

6   Bachevalier, J. and Loveland, K.A., 'The orbitofrontal–
    amygdala circuit and self-regulation of social–emotional
    behavior in autism', *Neuroscience & Biobehavioral Reviews*,
    2006, 30(1): p. 97–117.

7   Ressler, K.J., 'Amygdala activity, fear, and anxiety: modulation
    by stress', *Biological Psychiatry*, 2010, 67(12): p. 1117–19.

8   McLaughlin, K.A. and King, K., 'Developmental trajectories
    of anxiety and depression in early adolescence', *Journal of
    Abnormal Child Psychology*, 2015, 43(2): p. 311–23.

9   World Health Organization, 'Depression and other common
    mental disorders: global health estimates', 2017.

10 Lépine, J.-P., 'The epidemiology of anxiety disorders:
    prevalence and societal costs', *The Journal of Clinical
    Psychiatry*, 2002, 63 (Suppl 14): p. 4–8.

11 Cohen, D., *Sex, Gender, and Sexuality in Ancient Greece*, 1992,
    University of Chicago Press.

12 Hoge, E.A., Ivkovic, A., and Fricchione, G.L., 'Generalized
    anxiety disorder: diagnosis and treatment', *BMJ*, 2012, 345:
    p. e7500.

13 King, N.J., et al., 'Self-reports of panic attacks and manifest
    anxiety in adolescents', *Behaviour Research and Therapy*, 1993,
    31(1): p. 111–6.

14 Tull, M.T. and Roemer, L., 'Emotion regulation difficulties associated with the experience of uncued panic attacks: Evidence of experiential avoidance, emotional nonacceptance, and decreased emotional clarity', *Behavior Therapy*, 2007, 38(4): p. 378–91.

15 Milad, M.R., et al., 'Neurobiological basis of failure to recall extinction memory in posttraumatic stress disorder', *Biological Psychiatry*, 2009, 66(12): p. 1075–82.

16 Brewin, C.R., 'Memory processes in post-traumatic stress disorder', *International Review of Psychiatry*, 2001, 13(3): p. 159–63.

17 Peters, L., Slade, T., and Andrews, G., 'A comparison of ICD10 and DSM-IV criteria for posttraumatic stress disorder', *Journal of Traumatic Stress: Official Publication of The International Society for Traumatic Stress Studies*, 1999, 12(2): p. 335–43.

18 Baxter, A.J., et al., 'Global prevalence of anxiety disorders: a systematic review and meta-regression', *Psychological Medicine*, 2013, 43(5): p. 897–910.

19 Furmark, T., et al., 'Social phobia in the general population: prevalence and sociodemographic profile', *Social Psychiatry and Psychiatric Epidemiology*, 1999, 34(8): p. 416–24.

20 Flinn, M.V., Geary, D.C., and Ward, C.V., 'Ecological dominance, social competition, and coalitionary arms races: Why humans evolved extraordinary intelligence', *Evolution and Human Behavior*, 2005, 26(1): p. 10–46.

21 Woo, C.W., et al., 'Separate neural representations for physical pain and social rejection', *Nature Communications*, 2014, 5: p. 5380.

22 Bandelow, B., 'Comparison of the DSM-5 and ICD-10: panic and other anxiety disorders', *CNS Spectrums*, 2017, 22(5): p. 404–6.

23 Krzanowska, E. and Kuleta, M., 'From anxiety to compulsivity: a review of changes to OCD classification

in DSM-5 and ICD-11', *Archives of Psychiatry and Psychotherapy*, 2017, 19(3): p. 7–15.

24 Zorn, J.V., et al., 'Cortisol stress reactivity across psychiatric disorders: a systematic review and meta-analysis', *Psychoneuroendocrinology*, 2017, 77: p. 25–36.

25 McGowan, P.O. and Matthews, S.G., 'Prenatal stress, glucocorticoids, and developmental programming of the stress response', *Endocrinology*, 2018, 159(1): p. 69–82.

26 Stone, W.S., Rudd, R.J., and Gold, P.E., 'Amphetamine, epinephrine, and glucose enhancement of memory retrieval', *Psychobiology*, 1990, 18(2): p. 227–30.

27 Mezzacappa, E.S., 'Epinephrine, arousal, and emotion: A new look at two-factor theory', *Cognition and Emotion*, 1999, 13(2): p. 181–99.

28 Morales-Medina, J.C., Dumont, Y., and Quirion, R., 'A possible role of neuropeptide Y in depression and stress', *Brain Research*, 2010, 1314: p. 194–205.

29 Chen, H.Y., et al., 'Orexigenic action of peripheral ghrelin is mediated by neuropeptide Y and agouti-related protein', *Endocrinology*, 2004, 145(6): p. 2607–12.

30 Gold, A.L., Morey, R.A., and McCarthy, G., 'Amygdala–Prefrontal Cortex Functional Connectivity During Threat-Induced Anxiety and Goal Distraction', *Biological Psychiatry*, 2015, 77(4): p. 394–403.

31 Chebib, M. and Johnston, G.A., 'The "ABC" of GABA receptors: a brief review', *Clinical and Experimental Pharmacology and Physiology*, 1999, 26(11): p. 937–40.

32 Woodruff, A.R., Monyer, H., and Sah, P., 'GABAergic excitation in the basolateral amygdala', *The Journal of Neuroscience*, 2006, 26(46): p. 11881–7.

33 Delli Pizzi, S., et al., 'GABA content within the ventromedial prefrontal cortex is related to trait anxiety', *Social Cognitive and Affective Neuroscience*, 2016, 11(5): p. 758–66.

34 Nuss, P., 'Anxiety disorders and GABA neurotransmission: a disturbance of modulation', *Neuropsychiatric Disease and Treatment*, 2015, 11: p. 165–75.

35 Powers III, A.R., et al., 'Ketamine-induced hallucinations', *Psychopathology*, 2015, 48(6): p. 376–85.

36 Rune, G. and Frotscher, M., 'Neurosteroid synthesis in the hippocampus: role in synaptic plasticity', *Neuroscience*, 2005, 136(3): p. 833–42.

37 Hosie, A.M., et al., 'Endogenous neurosteroids regulate GABA A receptors through two discrete transmembrane sites', *Nature*, 2006, 444(7118): p. 486–9.

38 Gunn, B.G., et al., 'Neurosteroids and $GABA_A$ receptor interactions: a focus on stress', *Frontiers in Neuroscience*, 2011, 5: p. 131.

39 Stein, M.B., Jang, K.L., and Livesley, W.J., 'Heritability of anxiety sensitivity: a twin study', *American Journal of Psychiatry*, 1999, 156(2): p. 246–51.

40 Fareri, D.S. and Tottenham, N., 'Effects of early life stress on amygdala and striatal development', *Developmental Cognitive Neuroscience*, 2016, 19(Suppl C): p. 233–47.

41 Abelson, J.L., et al., 'HPA axis activity in patients with panic disorder: review and synthesis of four studies', *Depression and Anxiety*, 2007, 24(1): p. 66–76.

42 Pejic, T., et al., 'Social anxiety modulates amygdala activation during social conditioning', *Social Cognitive and Affective Neuroscience*, 2013, 8(3): p. 267–76.

43 Roth, G., 'The quest to find consciousness', *Scientific American Mind*, 2004, 14(1): p. 32–9.

44 Hawkins, K.A. and Cougle, J.R., 'Anger problems across the anxiety disorders: findings from a population-based study', *Depression and Anxiety*, 2011 28(2): p. 145–52.

45 Kapczinski, F., et al., 'Antidepressants for generalised anxiety disorder (GAD)', Cochrane Database of Systematic Reviews, 2003(2).

46 Cameron, O.G., 'Anxious-depressive comorbidity: effects on HPA axis and CNS noradrenergic functions', *Essential Psychopharmacology*, 2006, 7(1): p. 24–34.

47 Pinna, G., Costa, E., and Guidotti, A., 'SSRIs act as selective brain steroidogenic stimulants (SBSSs) at low doses that are inactive on 5-HT reuptake', *Current Opinion in Pharmacology*, 2009, 9(1): p. 24–30.

48 Pritchett, D.B., et al., 'Importance of a novel GABA A receptor subunit for benzodiazepine pharmacology', *Nature*, 1989, 338(6216): p. 582–85.

49 O'Brien, C.P., 'Benzodiazepine use, abuse, and dependence', *The Journal of Clinical Psychiatry*, 2005, 66 (Suppl 2): p. 28–33.

50 Foa, E.B., 'Prolonged exposure therapy: past, present, and future', *Depression and Anxiety*, 2011, 28(12): p. 1043–7.

51 Clark, D., 'The treatment of monosymptomatic phobia by systematic desensitization', *Behaviour Research and Therapy*, 1963, 1(1): p. 63–8.

52 Gauvreau, P. and Bouchard, S., 'Preliminary evidence for the efficacy of EMDR in treating generalized anxiety disorder', *Journal of EMDR Practice and Research*, 2008, 2(1): p. 26–40.

5: Addiction

1 Drake, R.E., Mueser, K.T., and Brunette, M.F., 'Management of persons with co-occurring severe mental illness and substance

use disorder: program implications', *World Psychiatry: Official Journal of the World Psychiatric Association (WPA)*, 2007, 6(3): p. 131–36.

2   Budney, A.J., et al., 'Caffeine withdrawal and dependence: a convenience survey among addiction professionals', *Journal of Caffeine Research*, 2013, 3(2): p. 67–71.

3   Hawkes, C.H., 'Endorphins: the basis of pleasure?', *Journal of Neurology, Neurosurgery and Psychiatry*, 1992, 55(4): p. 247–50.

4   Koob, G.F., 'A role for GABA mechanisms in the motivational effects of alcohol', *Biochemical Pharmacology*, 2004, 68(8): p. 1515–25.

5   Gardner, E.L., 'Introduction: Addiction and Brain Reward and Anti-Reward Pathways', *Advances in Psychosomatic Medicine*, 2011, 30: p. 22–60.

6   Parkinson Study Group, 'Levodopa and the progression of Parkinson's disease', *New England Journal of Medicine*, 2004, 351(24): p. 2498–508.

7   Pietrzykowski, A.Z. and Treistman, S.N., 'The molecular basis of tolerance', *Alcohol Research & Health: The Journal of the National Institute on Alcohol Abuse and Alcoholism*, 2008, 31(4): p. 298–309.

8   Kalivas, P.W. and Volkow, N.D., 'The neural basis of addiction: a pathology of motivation and choice', *American Journal of Psychiatry*, 2005, 162(8): p. 1403–13.

9   Dickinson, A. and Mackintosh, N., 'Classical conditioning in animals', *Annual Review of Psychology*, 1978, 29(1): p. 587–612.

10 Koob, G.F. and Franz, K.J., 'The neurobiology of addiction', in Holman Coombs, R. (ed.), *Addiction Counseling Review* (Routledge, 2004): p. 57–82.

11 Darke, S., Larney, S., and Farrell, M., 'Yes, people can die from opiate withdrawal', *Addiction*, 2017, 112(2): p. 199–200.

12 Hartmann-Boyce, J., et al., 'Electronic cigarettes for smoking cessation', Cochrane Database of Systematic Reviews, 2016(9).

13 Grant, J.E. and Chamberlain, S.R., 'Expanding the definition of addiction: DSM-5 vs. ICD-11', *CNS Spectrums*, 2016, 21(4): p. 300–3.

14 Musalek, M., 'Pathological gambling: Addiction or impulse control disorder', *European Psychiatry*, 2007, 22(S1): p. S37.

15 Carnes, P.J., 'Addiction or compulsion: politics or illness?', *Sexual Addiction & Compulsivity: The Journal of Treatment and Prevention*, 1996, 3(2): p. 127–150.

16 Panova, T. and Carbonell, X., 'Is smartphone addiction really an addiction?', *Journal of Behavioral Addictions*, 2018, 7(2): p. 252–9.

17 Papageorgiou, C., et al., 'Do obsessive-compulsive patients and abstinent heroin addicts share a common psychophysiological mechanism?', *Neuropsychobiology*, 2003, 47(1): p. 1–11.

18 DiClemente, C.C. and Prochaska, J.O., 'Toward a comprehensive, transtheoretical model of change: Stages of change and addictive behaviors', in W. R. Miller & N. Heather (Eds.), *Applied clinical psychology. Treating addictive behaviors* (1998, Plenum Press): p. 3–24.

19 O'Brien, C.P., Volkow, N., and Li, T., 'What's in a word? Addiction versus dependence in DSM-V', *The American Journal of Psychiatry*, 2006 163(5): 764–5.

20 Agrawal, A., et al., 'The genetics of addiction – a translational perspective', *Translational Psychiatry*, 2012, 2(7): p. e140.

21 Patoine, B., 'Desperately Seeking Sensation: Fear, Reward, and the Human Need for Novelty', The Dana Foundation, 2009.

Conclusion

1 Kiecolt-Glaser, J.K., Derry, H.M., and Fagundes, C.P., 'Inflammation: Depression Fans the Flames and Feasts on the Heat', *American Journal of Psychiatry*, 2015, 172(11): p. 1075–91.